NO GODS, NO GURUS

NO GODS, NO GURUS

A Radical Guide to
Your Well-Being

DR NANDITA IYER

BLOOMSBURY
NEW DELHI · LONDON · OXFORD · NEW YORK · SYDNEY

BLOOMSBURY INDIA
Bloomsbury Publishing India Pvt. Ltd
Second Floor, LSC Building No. 4, DDA Complex, Pocket C – 6 & 7,
Vasant Kunj, New Delhi, 110070

BLOOMSBURY, BLOOMSBURY INDIA and the Diana logo
are trademarks of Bloomsbury Publishing Plc

First published in India 2025

Copyright © Dr Nandita Iyer, 2025

Dr Nandita Iyer has asserted her moral rights to be identified as the author
of this work in accordance with the Indian Copyright Act, 1957

The views and opinions expressed in this book are the author's own and
the publisher is in no way liable for the same

Some names and details of individuals have been changed to preserve their anonymity

This book is not a substitute for medical attention, treatment, examination, advice,
treatment of existing conditions or diagnosis. It is not intended to provide a clinical
diagnosis nor take the place of medical advice from a fully qualified medical
practitioner. Consult your healthcare service provider before following any
health advice given in this book

All rights reserved. No part of this publication may be: i) reproduced or transmitted
in any form, electronic or mechanical, including photocopying, recording or by
means of any information storage or retrieval system without prior permission in
writing from the publishers; or ii) used or reproduced in any way for the training,
development or operation of artificial intelligence (AI) technologies, including
generative AI technologies. The rights holders expressly reserve this publication from
the text and data mining exception as per Article 4(3) of the Digital Single Market
Directive (EU) 2019/790

ISBN: PB: 9789361319570; eBook: 9789361319679
2 4 6 8 10 9 7 5 3 1

Typeset in Minion by Manipal Technologies Limited
Printed and bound in India by Thomson Press India Ltd

To find out more about our authors and books visit www.bloomsbury.com and sign
up for our newsletters

To Amma and my aunts, Geeta, Prabha, and Revathi, who wear their seventies (and late sixties) with quiet strength, youthfulness, and grace. Their simple, disciplined lives, built on years of hard work, resilience, and spirituality, have shaped me into the person I am today.

Contents

PART I	The Foundations	1
PART II	Food, Fad, and Fiction	61
PART III	Built to Move	139
PART IV	Your Home, Your Health	169
PART V	The Hormone Connection	197
PART VI	Sleep: The Missing Superpower	227
PART VII	Mind Matters	245
PART VIII	Living Long, Living Well	285

Acknowledgements	301
Notes	303
About the Author	311

Part I

The Foundations

1. Decoding the True Indicators of Good Health
2. The Power of Metabolic Flexibility
3. Inflammation: The Hidden Roadblock to Health (and Weight Loss)
4. Nurturing Your Immune System
5. How to Keep Your Heart Ticking for Long
6. Is It Possible to Detox Your Liver?
7. Microbiome Matters: Decoding Gut Health
8. Activate Your Inner Calm: The Vagus Nerve Guide
9. The Great Energy Heist
10. Making Fat Loss Happen: A Real-World Manual
11. Fad-Proof Your Health
12. Health Check-Ups: Your Annual Power Move
13. Genetic Testing: The Truth Behind the Trend

Part I

The Foundations

1

Decoding the True Indicators of Good Health

The alarm breaks the silence, giving a jarring summons to the day.

Your eyes jolt open. Before your mind kicks in, your body tells you how it feels. Are you rising from a deep, restful sleep, alert and ready? Or are you dragging yourself into the morning, already tired? That first moment, before you check your phone or reach for coffee, is your body's unfiltered report card.

Think of your heart as the command centre of your body. With each heartbeat, it sends messages. Is it calm and steady or always in a rush to keep up with life? Your blood pressure tells its own story. It is a measure of how flexible your arteries are and how easily your heart moves blood through them. When it stays steady and within normal limits, it's a sign that your cardiovascular system is in good shape and managing life's demands with ease.

Your blood carries glucose and lipids, among other things. When your blood sugar and cholesterol are within a healthy range, your body feels balanced and energetic, while lingering sugars or rogue triglycerides sound warning bells.

After climbing a flight of stairs, notice how quickly your elevated heart rate slows again. Ideally, it should drop by about 12 beats in a minute. This heart rate recovery is your resilience score – the speed at which your body returns to its resting state.

Grip a doorknob firmly. That strength in your hand is a clue to your future vitality.

Sit on the floor and then stand up without using your hands. This simple act combines strength, balance, flexibility, and neuromuscular coordination. Surprisingly, the ease or difficulty in doing it can predict your mortality risk with remarkable precision.

It is bedtime. Do you fall asleep easily and wake up refreshed, or do you lie awake, with your mind spinning?

Energy is the central thread of your daily life. Does it flow evenly or often crash and spike, dragging your focus and mood with it? Those patterns reveal how smoothly your metabolism switches between fuel sources.

Your digestion is another piece of the story. After meals, do you feel comfortable and satisfied or bloated and uneasy? Your gut is an entire ecosystem, influencing immunity, hormones, and even mood. When it runs smoothly, so does everything else.

For women, monthly rhythms reveal additional insights. Regular cycles reflect hormonal balance and stable energy. When the inner system is in tune, it shows on the outside – clear skin, strong nails, and good mood.

Can you easily recall someone's name or master new skills? Whether your mind is sharp or foggy reflects your neurological health.

If life were a movie, your emotional state would be the background music. Is it mostly harmonious or full of noise and static? Your emotional state mirrors the balance of your hormones and nervous system more than you realise.

I am taking you through this guided tour of your body's landscape because we have lost our way. Modern medicine excels in crisis intervention but often misses these subtle yet powerful indicators that can predict the onset of a disease years or decades before it develops. Meanwhile, the wellness industry sells oversimplified solutions without helping you understand your unique biology.

Your body never stops communicating. It conveys a wealth of information through sensations, functions, limitations, and capacities. Its language is more precise and personalised than any generic health advice. Learning to interpret these signals is your trusted path to true well-being.

When we begin to decode these signals – physical, emotional, and everything in between – they lead us to the five dimensions that make up true health.

The Five Core Principles

Health exists in five interconnected dimensions, each revealing a different facet of your well-being:

Physical strength and function

True physical health goes beyond appearance or weight; it is reflected in how well your body functions. A strong grip correlates with a longer lifespan and better overall strength. The ability to get up from the floor without using hands for support (sit-to-stand test) and overall coordination says more about your biological age than any lab report. Carrying groceries, lifting objects, doing household tasks with ease, and walking up a flight of stairs without getting winded reflect your mobility and strength and indicate how your body handles exertion.

Mental agility

How quickly you think, react, and make decisions, as well as how well you learn and retain information, are all reflections of your brain's health. But cognitive fitness is more than just memory. It is also about clarity, focus, and the ability to remain mentally present without a constant haze or brain fog – common issues in today's hyperconnected world. Even before blood tests reveal signs of accelerated ageing, your mind may show the first clues.

Emotional balance

Are you able to overcome life's challenges while keeping a positive outlook? Your emotional landscape is a crucial dimension of your health. It is a reflection of the stability of your mood, your ability to process feelings without being overwhelmed, and your capacity for appropriate responses to life's challenges. Balanced moods are linked to regulated stress hormones, stable blood sugar, and a robust immune system.

Social connection

Humans evolved to thrive in a community, rather than in isolation. Strong social ties do not just feel good; they also lower inflammation, boost longevity, and act as emotional buffers in stressful times. In a country where family ties still matter, but loneliness is creeping in through the cracks of modern life, this dimension of health needs special attention.

Spiritual anchor

A sense of meaning, whether through faith, purpose, or connection to something greater than yourself, holds everything together. It encompasses the profound realisation that your life matters, that you are part of something enduring, whether that is a community, the natural world, a higher power, or a creative calling.

These five core principles do not operate in isolation. Neglect one, and the rest will falter. Nourish one, and all will thrive. That is the essence and challenge of achieving true holistic health.

Your Health, Your Way

Health is not one-size-fits-all. It's shaped by your genes, your age, your environment, and your daily choices. A 25-year-old and a 60-year-old have different goals; a city dweller and a farmer live under different kinds of stress. Your diet, stress levels, and sleep patterns all shape your health in ways that generic advice often overlooks.

Moreover, health is not static. It ebbs and flows with your life's chapters. That is why you need to check in with yourself often. How is your energy? How is your mood? How well do you bounce back? The answers are more revealing than any annual check-up.

The Ripple Effect

Visualise this: You begin walking daily (physical activity). Your stamina increases, which boosts your mood (emotional well-being). You work with more focus (mental clarity), call an old friend (social connection), and journal the things you are grateful for that day (spiritual growth). One small shift sends ripples through every layer of health.

Of course, the reverse is true too. Chronic stress raises cortisol, disturbs sleep, dulls joy, and unsettles everything else.

As we move through this book together, you will learn to notice these patterns, catch the early warnings, celebrate the small wins, and understand what truly matters for your body.

You will move beyond numbers and begin to understand what real health feels like.

Putting It into Practice

- **Rate yourself**: Score each core principle (on a scale of 1 to 10). Where do you need improvement?

- **Make one move**: Choose an area. Swap sugary coffee for black coffee or herbal tea (physical), doodle your thoughts (mental), or call a loved one (social).

You've Got This

Let us look at health as a free-flowing conversation between your body and your choices. When you learn to listen deeply, you begin to uncover a definition of health that is radically your own.

2

The Power of Metabolic Flexibility

Ashwin, a 35-year-old software engineer, was worried about his expanding waistline and constant fatigue. Climbing the corporate ladder meant longer hours at his desk, irregular meals, and minimal physical activity. Like many, he did not realise that his body had lost the ability to switch efficiently between energy sources, a key sign of poor metabolic flexibility.

Metabolic flexibility is a concept that is gaining popularity, and it is worth understanding.

What Exactly Is Metabolic Flexibility?

Metabolic flexibility refers to the body's ability to adapt to different available fuel sources, easily switching between glucose and fat. Think of it as a hybrid car. After eating a meal rich in carbs, a metabolically flexible person efficiently uses glucose for energy. However, during an overnight fast or between meals, they rely on stored body fats to maintain energy levels without crashing or getting 'hangry'.

Our hunter-gatherer ancestors naturally had this flexibility. They did not have regular access to food or the convenience of instant delivery of late-night snacks. Their bodies were adapted to switching to fat burning in the absence of food. In contrast, modern lifestyles, characterised by constant eating, sedentary habits, processed foods, and poor sleep, have led many people to lose this metabolic flexibility. Most of us with the privilege of having food available at any time of the day or night have forgotten what hunger really feels like. This makes the body depend on glucose for energy at all times, leading to frequent hunger pangs, low energy levels, stubborn weight gain, and insulin resistance.

Signs of Poor Metabolic Flexibility

Take this quiz

If your answer to many of the following questions is 'yes', then your metabolic flexibility may need overhauling:
- Do you become irritable or tired if you skip a meal?
- Do you feel hungry shortly after eating?
- Do you constantly crave sugar or refined carbs?
- Do you struggle to lose weight despite eating 'healthy'?
- Do you rely on caffeine or snacks to get through the day?
- Do you feel exhausted after light activity?

These are all signs that your body struggles to tap into fat as fuel and is overly dependent on glucose.

The Benefits of Having Metabolic Flexibility

- Metabolically flexible people can go longer between meals without experiencing energy crashes, irritability, or brain fog, and they maintain stable energy throughout the day.
- When your body can efficiently burn stored fat, it supports weight management and reduces stores of visceral fat (the harmful type linked to heart disease and diabetes).
- Being able to switch between burning glucose and fat allows for sustained endurance, improved performance, and better recovery after workouts.
- Good metabolic flexibility is a sign of strong insulin sensitivity. This means your body does not overproduce insulin, helping to prevent type 2 diabetes.
- A lack of metabolic flexibility is linked to chronic low-grade inflammation, fatty liver, polycystic ovary syndrome (PCOS), and metabolic syndrome.
- A flexible metabolism supports mitochondrial health (your cellular energy engines), which plays a significant role in how well we age.

How Do We Go Wrong?

Several lifestyle factors can sabotage your metabolic flexibility. Some of them are as follows:
- A sedentary lifestyle

- Ultra-processed, high-carb diets
- Constant snacking or grazing
- Poor sleep and high stress levels
- Insulin resistance or prediabetes
- Over-reliance on carbs while underusing fat for energy

All these factors 'de-train' your metabolism from using fat as a fuel source, keeping you hooked on sugar-burning mode. A regular diet high in refined carbs and sugar leads to glucose dominance and insulin resistance. Additionally, sedentary behaviour reduces the need to tap into fat stores for energy. Poor sleep and chronic stress affect hormone regulation and energy metabolism.

How to Retrain and Regain Your Metabolic Flexibility

The good news is that you can improve poor metabolic flexibility, and your body responds surprisingly well, even if you have experienced years of sluggish metabolism, insulin resistance, or a dependence on frequent eating.

With the right strategies, your body can relearn how to switch between using glucose (sugar) and fat as fuel more efficiently. Metabolic flexibility is trainable, just like physical fitness. So let us explore the steps you can take to train it.

The evidence-backed strategies for regaining flexibility fall into three categories, and no prizes for guessing that these are diet, exercise, and lifestyle changes.

Diet

- Reducing overall carbohydrate intake, especially refined carbohydrates and sugars, encourages your body to become more efficient at burning fat for fuel.
- Focus on a diet that is rich in whole, unprocessed foods. Prioritise fibre-rich vegetables, with moderate portions of whole grains, lentils, and legumes, and include fruit in controlled amounts. This approach helps stabilise blood sugar levels and enhances insulin sensitivity, both key components of metabolic flexibility. Dietary fibre slows the absorption of glucose, preventing sharp spikes and crashes in blood sugar.
- Avoid frequent snacking, giving your body windows to utilise stored fat for energy. Start with a 12-hour overnight fast and

gradually increase to 14–15 hours over a few weeks if you find it manageable.
- While a ketogenic diet is known to improve the body's ability to use fat as the primary energy source, it may not be a sustainable long-term strategy for everyone.

Exercise

- Aerobic workouts (such as running, swimming, or cycling) enhance mitochondrial function and fat oxidation, which are important for effective fuel switching.
- Resistance training builds muscle, improving insulin sensitivity and glucose management.
- HIIT (high-intensity interval training) boosts both glucose and fat metabolism efficiently.
- A combination of cardio and strength training delivers the best metabolic flexibility benefits.

Lifestyle

Beyond diet and exercise, other lifestyle factors also play a role.
- Getting adequate, quality sleep is essential for metabolic health. Sleep deprivation can disrupt hormones that regulate appetite and glucose metabolism, potentially leading to metabolic inflexibility. Aim for seven to nine hours of quality sleep every night.
- Chronic stress can lead to hormonal imbalances that negatively impact metabolism and blood sugar control. Implementing stress-management techniques such as meditation, yoga, or spending time in nature can be beneficial.
- Prolonged sitting has been associated with metabolic inflexibility, even in individuals who meet physical activity recommendations. Breaking up long periods of sitting with short bouts of movement throughout the day can help improve metabolic health.

While it is not always necessary, assessing metabolic flexibility can provide valuable insights into your current metabolic state and help track progress. Your doctor can choose from various methods, including laboratory-based techniques or at-home devices. Some wearables, like the Apple Watch, track heart rate variability (HRV), which can indicate metabolic health. Higher HRV is generally associated with better metabolic flexibility. A handheld device (Lumen) aims to measure your body's current fuel utilisation based on breath carbon dioxide analysis. It uses this data to provide a 'Flex Score' that reflects your metabolic flexibility over time. It then offers personalised advice to help improve this aspect of your metabolic health.

Putting It into Practice

- Try a twelve-hour overnight fast for one week. For example, finish dinner by 8 p.m. and eat breakfast after 8 a.m. See how your energy levels respond during this time.
- Incorporate two to three sessions of low-intensity cardio (like walking or cycling) while on an empty stomach. This trains your body to use fat as fuel.

You've Got This

Metabolic flexibility is more than a buzzword. It is a powerful reflection of how well your body can adapt, survive, and thrive. Like fitness or strength, it is entirely trainable, and the benefits extend beyond weight loss. Better energy, sharper focus, and improved hormone balance are just a few consistent steps away.

3

Inflammation: The Hidden Roadblock to Health (and Weight Loss)

In October 2024, a video featuring actor Vidya Balan went viral.[1] She was not peddling detox teas, flaunting a 30-day challenge, or blaming carbs for weight gain. Instead, she was explaining that her recent weight loss was not due to starving herself or 'doing cardio like crazy', but from switching to an anti-inflammatory diet. The internet broke into a frenzy: 'What is this magical anti-inflammatory diet?', 'Is inflammation the reason I am not losing weight?', 'Is this legit or just another wellness buzzword?'

Before we start looking at gluten as a villain and adding turmeric to every meal in the hope of cutting out inflammation, let us ask a more useful question: what exactly is inflammation and should you be concerned about it?

Your Body's Fire Alarm System

Inflammation is your immune system's response to injury, infection, or threat. It is similar to a firefighter rushing in when your body sends out an SOS.

Did you cut your finger? The redness and swelling indicate that white blood cells are at work. Caught a cold? The fever and fatigue signal that your body is gearing up to fight off the illness. Feeling sore after a workout? That sensation is due to healing inflammation.

This type of inflammation is acute inflammation – it is short-term, targeted, and essential. Once the job is done, it dials down.

When Inflammation Becomes a Problem

Inflammation itself is not the villain; the issue is chronic inflammation. It is like a low-grade fire smouldering beneath the surface. Although it may not produce noticeable symptoms, it contributes to heart disease, diabetes, PCOS, autoimmune conditions, Alzheimer's disease, obesity, and even cancer.

Chronic inflammation is fuelled by poor diet, stress, lack of physical activity, inadequate sleep, and toxins. The good news is that you can reverse it.

What Are the Signs of Chronic Inflammation?

The signs of chronic inflammation are subtle and progress gradually, such that many times your body simply takes it in its stride, and it becomes the new normal for you, until the symptoms become hard to ignore. Here are some of the red flags to watch for:
- Constant fatigue
- Brain fog
- Digestive issues, such as bloating or irritable bowel syndrome
- Skin breakouts or rashes
- Joint pain or stiffness
- Frequent infections or slow recovery
- Unexplained weight gain or difficulty losing weight

Even if you feel 'mostly okay', chronic inflammation might be simmering beneath the surface, setting the stage for future health issues.

What Causes Chronic Inflammation?

A few major drivers of chronic inflammation are as follows:
- Consumption of ultra-processed foods (UPFs)
- A sedentary lifestyle that reduces circulation and metabolic rate
- Poor sleep, which disrupts immune regulation and increases stress hormones
- Chronic stress, which keeps cortisol levels elevated and the immune response on overdrive
- Excess body fat, especially visceral fat, which itself is inflammatory

- Unaddressed infections or gut imbalances like dysbiosis or leaky gut
- Environmental toxins from pollution, plastics, and pesticides

In short, a modern lifestyle can set the stage for chronic inflammation. However, it does not mean we are doomed.

The level of inflammation in the body can be measured by blood tests, including:
- hs-CRP (high-sensitivity C-reactive protein)
- ESR (erythrocyte sedimentation rate)
- Fibrinogen
- Interleukins, TNF-alpha (advanced)

These tests are not routine, but if you experience fatigue, hormonal issues, or stubborn weight, consult your doctor.

An Anti-Inflammatory Lifestyle

Reducing inflammation in the body requires lifestyle changes and, in some cases, medical intervention. Here are evidence-based steps you can take:
- **Eat anti-inflammatory foods**: Focus on whole foods, leafy greens, fish, nuts, olive oil, and whole grains. Avoid processed foods, sugar, red meat, and alcohol. Add turmeric and ginger to your diet.
- **Exercise regularly**: Aim for 150 minutes of moderate or 75 minutes of vigorous exercise per week, along with strength training. Do not overtrain, as this can also increase inflammation.
- **Manage stress**: Practise mindfulness, meditation, yoga, or deep breathing to lower cortisol levels and reduce inflammatory markers. Chronic stress can trigger inflammation, so it is essential to prioritise relaxation.
- **Get adequate sleep**: Aim for seven to nine hours of quality sleep nightly. Poor sleep increases inflammatory cytokines.
- **Maintain a healthy weight**: Excess body fat, especially visceral fat, promotes inflammation. Gradual weight loss through diet and exercise can help.
- **Quit smoking and alcohol**: Smoking increases systemic inflammation, but quitting can reduce it over time. Limit alcohol

to moderate levels (one drink per day for women and two for men). However, the best option is to quit alcohol completely.
- **Stay hydrated**: Drink adequate water daily (about eight to ten glasses, depending on your activity level and the climate) to support cellular function and help reduce inflammation.
- **Consider supplements**: Omega-3 fish oil, curcumin, or vitamin D may be beneficial, but consult your doctor before starting any supplements, as they can interact with medications. Do not rely solely on supplements without making dietary changes.
- **Manage chronic conditions**: Work with your doctor to control conditions like diabetes, arthritis, or autoimmune diseases that can drive inflammation. Follow prescribed treatments.
- **Avoid environmental triggers**: Minimise exposure to pollutants, allergens, or irritants (such as air pollution and mould) that can trigger inflammation. Use air purifiers or wear masks in high-pollution areas if needed.

Together, these changes can lower inflammatory markers like CRP and improve overall well-being.

Putting It into Practice

- Tune in to symptoms like fatigue or bloating – your body might be asking for help.
- Audit your food, stress, and sleep to identify triggers you can change.

You've Got This

You do not need a trendy label or a celebrity endorsement to reduce inflammation. What you need is consistency, real food, deep rest, and the wisdom to stop fighting your body and start supporting it.

Vidya's story lit a spark. Now it is your turn to take action.

4

Nurturing Your Immune System

If the world learned anything from the COVID-19 pandemic, it was that we knew far less about our immune systems than we thought. While governments scrambled to communicate hygiene protocols, a parallel surge unfolded online. Suddenly, everyone became an amateur immunologist. *Kaadhas* (potions made with an array of spices) were rebranded as immunity elixirs. Grandma's *haldi doodh* went viral. Shelves were running out of vitamin C, zinc, and *chyawanprash* and Google searches for 'immune system' and 'vitamin C' spiked. A survery conducted in August 2020 revealed that 60 per cent of the adult users of dietary supplements had increased their multivitamin supplement routine.[2]

However, immunity is far more nuanced than simply popping supplements or sipping turmeric lattes.

The immune system is not a single organ that can be 'boosted' on demand. In fact, the very concept of boosting immunity is scientifically misleading. An overactive immune system can lead to autoimmune diseases and chronic inflammation. What we really need is an immune system that is balanced, adaptable, and resilient – neither sluggish nor hyperactive, but intelligently responsive.

This chapter will not offer miracle foods or magic pills. Instead, we will explore the simple, often overlooked choices that contribute to immune health over time. The kind of advice that rarely goes viral but quietly builds long-term resilience.

Your Inner Defence Force: A Quick Refresher

The immune system is a complex network of organs, cells, and proteins that protects the body from infections, toxins, and abnormal or damaged cells. It includes components such as white blood cells, the lymphatic system, bone marrow, the thymus, as well as the skin and gut lining. The innate immune system responds quickly and broadly, while the adaptive immune system develops memory and precision over time.

Both systems thrive on balanced inputs via nutrition, sleep, stress management, and microbial exposure. Unfortunately, modern lifestyles, with processed diets, sleepless nights, chronic stress, and sterile environments, rarely provide these inputs in the right balance.

Do Supplements Work?

The pandemic sparked a rush for quick-fix solutions, with many supplements marketed as immunity shields. But can a pill or powder truly transform your defences? Let us explore the hype and focus on what really works.

Supplements can help support immunity by addressing specific deficiencies but are no substitute for lifestyle interventions. For instance, vitamin D can reduce respiratory infection risk in individuals who are deficient, while vitamin C may shorten cold duration. Zinc can lessen cold severity, probiotics can lower respiratory infection rates, and elderberry may ease viral symptoms. However, these are most effective when tailored to specific needs, and overuse can lead to side effects such as toxicity. Consult a doctor to assess deficiencies instead of relying on marketed 'immune blends'. Be wary of products that make vague claims, as regulation is often lax in the supplement industry and evidence of their effectiveness in improving immunity remains limited.

Beyond Supplements: A Holistic Framework

While supplements like vitamin D or probiotics may support immunity in specific contexts, they are not a panacea. The immune system flourishes on a range of interconnected lifestyle factors that require consistent attention.

Nutrition plays the role of the engine

A nutrient-dense diet is the central pillar of immune health. The immune system relies on vitamins (A, C, D, E), minerals (zinc and selenium), and phytonutrients in whole foods. For example, a 2019

study linked diets rich in fruits and vegetables to enhanced T-cell function, which is critical for fighting infections.[2] To enhance your immune health, consider incorporating the following foods in your diet:
- Colourful produce, such as mango, amla, pomegranate, guava, leafy greens, and orange vegetables, which provide antioxidants that combat oxidative stress.
- Healthy fats, such as omega-3 fatty acids in salmon and walnuts, that reduce inflammation.
- Fermented foods, such as yoghurt, kombucha, tempeh, and kimchi, which support gut microbiota.

Additionally, it is important to avoid processed foods high in sugar and trans fats, as these can impair immune signalling.

Sleep resets your immune system

Sleep is non-negotiable for immunity. During sleep, the body produces cytokines, which are proteins that help regulate immune responses. A 2015 study found that getting less than seven hours of sleep each night increases susceptibility to viral infections by 30 per cent.[4] To support better sleep, focus on the following:
- A consistent sleep schedule
- A dark, cool environment in the bedroom
- Limiting screen time before bed to enhance melatonin production

Importance of physical activity

Moderate exercise bolsters immunity by promoting circulation and reducing chronic inflammation. A 2021 review reported that 150 minutes of weekly moderate aerobic activity (e.g., brisk walking) enhances the body's antibody response to vaccines.[5] However, it is important to note that excessive exercise can suppress immunity, so it is best to avoid overtraining.

Stress management

Chronic stress elevates cortisol levels, which suppresses immune cell activity. A 2020 study linked high stress to a reduction in natural killer cell function.[6] Practices such as mindfulness, yoga, or deep breathing can reduce stress levels. Even 20 minutes of daily meditation has been found to improve immune markers in adults.[7]

Social connection

Human connection influences immunity via the gut-brain axis. A 2019 study[8] revealed that strong social ties are associated with lower inflammation markers. Engaging in meaningful relationships and participating in community activities can help boost your immune system's resilience.

The Not-So-Obvious Factors

Shaping immunity in early life

Immune resilience begins at birth. Several factors influence long-term immune strength, including being born via vaginal delivery (which exposes the newborn to the maternal microbiome), being breastfed (which provides antibodies and immune-supportive compounds like lactoferrin), and exposure to diverse microbes in early childhood. The 'hygiene hypothesis' suggests that overly sanitised environments may hinder immune development, making us more prone to allergies and autoimmune conditions.

Environmental toxins

- Pollution, endocrine-disrupting chemicals (such as BPA or Bisphenol A and phthalates), and microplastics can disrupt immune function.
- Air pollution, in particular, heightens the risk of respiratory infections.
- BPA and phthalates (commonly found in plastics and personal care products) can impair immune signalling. Reducing exposure to these toxins can support immune health.

The gut-immune axis

Around 70–80 per cent of immune activity occurs in the gut. The trillions of microbes living there help educate immune cells, manage inflammation, and teach the body to distinguish friend from foe. Yet most urban Indian diets, low in fibre and high in processed food, are not good for the microbiome. Increasing your intake of fermented foods (e.g., yoghurt, idli, or dhokla), prebiotics (e.g., raw bananas, garlic, onions), and fibre-rich vegetables (e.g., bhindi, spinach) is one of the most effective ways to support immunity at the source.[9]

Putting It into Practice

- Include a variety of colourful fruits, vegetables, and lentils in your daily meals.
- Develop good sleep habits and ensure you get seven to eight hours of quality sleep each night.
- Move your body regularly, but do not overdo it.
- Incorporate simple stress-reduction tools into your daily routine.

You've Got This

The post-COVID obsession with immunity highlighted both our vulnerability and our capacity for proactive health. While brands profited from fear-driven marketing, scientific evidence points to a broader truth that immunity is a lifestyle, not a product. Let us move beyond quick fixes to sustainable practices that empower us to thrive in an unpredictable world, without being sold yet another 'immunity-boosting' product.

5
How to Keep Your Heart Ticking for Long

You do not notice your heart until there is a problem. It pumps over 7,500 litres of blood every day without asking for a break, yet most of us treat it like a background app, running silently while we binge on sugar, take stress, and increase our screen time.

We are well aware that heart attacks do not always wait for old age. They are showing up earlier, often in people who 'look healthy'. Fortunately, the heart is forgiving. With a few powerful changes in how you move, eat, and live, you can cut your risk dramatically and give your body's most loyal muscle the support it deserves. Whether you are 25 or 65, now is the time to pay attention. Let us dive into practical, heart-healthy habits that will keep your ticker strong for years to come.

Food for a Healthy Heart

Poor nutrition is one of the leading global causes of heart disease, but it is also one of the easiest issues to improve. A balanced, heart-healthy diet has a powerful and measurable impact on key risk factors. It can lower low-density lipoprotein (LDL) cholesterol, reduce blood pressure and inflammation, and support healthy blood vessels. Here are some ways to nourish your heart through food:
- **Focus on healthy fats**: Healthy fats, particularly unsaturated fats, are vital for heart health. Sources include avocados, nuts, seeds, cold-pressed oils like mustard, groundnut, extra virgin olive oil, or even homemade ghee in moderation. If you eat fish, consider adding fatty varieties like mackerel (bangda), which are rich in heart-protective omega-3s. These fats help reduce levels of LDL, which is associated with plaque build-up in arteries, and increase HDL (high-density lipoprotein), which

supports cholesterol clearance from the bloodstream – thereby lowering cardiovascular risk.
- **Fibre-rich foods**: Fibre, especially soluble fibre, plays a crucial role in reducing cholesterol and promoting heart health. Foods high in fibre include whole grains (like oats, barley, quinoa), legumes (beans, lentils, chickpeas), fruits (apples, pears, guava), and vegetables (broccoli, carrots, spinach). A high-fibre diet can also help manage blood sugar levels, which is important for preventing heart disease.
- **Lean protein**: Protein is essential for building and repairing tissues, but the type of protein you consume matters. Choose lean protein sources such as chicken, fish, tofu, and legumes (not the best sources of protein), while limiting red meat and processed meats. These can increase the risk of heart disease due to their saturated fat content.
- **Limit added sugars and refined carbs**: Consuming excessive amounts of added sugars and refined carbohydrates can lead to weight gain, increased inflammation, and higher triglyceride levels, all of which can negatively affect heart health. Instead, opt for whole grains like brown rice and whole wheat, and limit (or avoid) sugary snacks, sodas, and processed foods.
- **Antioxidants and anti-inflammatory foods**: Foods rich in antioxidants, such as amla, leafy greens, and nuts, help fight oxidative stress and inflammation, both of which can contribute to heart disease. Incorporating a variety of colourful fruits and vegetables into your diet provides essential vitamins and minerals to keep your heart healthy.

Exercise, the Heart's Best Ally

Exercise comes a close second to food as a critical factor in improving heart function.

Physical activity is one of the most effective ways to maintain heart health. Regular exercise helps strengthen the heart muscle, improve circulation, and regulate essential metrics such as blood pressure, cholesterol, and blood sugar. The heart, like any other muscle, becomes stronger and more efficient with regular exercise.
- **Aerobic exercise**: Activities like walking, jogging, cycling, and swimming that elevate your heart rate are examples of aerobic

exercise. Aim for at least 150 minutes of moderate-intensity exercise per week or 75 minutes of vigorous-intensity activity. This could be split into 30-minute sessions on most days of the week, making it easy to incorporate into your daily routine.
- **Strength training**: In addition to aerobic exercise, strength training plays a critical role in heart health. Building muscle mass helps improve metabolism, regulate blood sugar, and reduce fat, thereby reducing the strain on your heart. For heart health, you do not need to lift heavy weights. Simple bodyweight exercises like squats, lunges, and push-ups can be just as effective. Aim to incorporate strength training into your routine at least twice a week.
- **Flexibility and balance**: Practices such as yoga, Pilates, and tai chi may not get your heart rate soaring, but they still contribute to heart health by improving flexibility, reducing stress, and supporting healthy circulation. Additionally, they help with balance and posture, which can reduce the risk of falls and injuries, especially as we age.
- **Interval training**: If time is a constraint, HIIT offers a highly efficient way to improve heart health. HIIT involves alternating between intense bursts of activity and rest periods, which challenge your cardiovascular system and burn fat more effectively. This method can deliver significant heart health benefits in a short amount of time, making it an excellent choice for busy individuals.

Lifestyle Habits

In addition to exercise and nutrition, your lifestyle choices play a critical role in maintaining a healthy heart. Stress management, quality sleep, and avoiding harmful habits can all help protect your heart and improve its function.
- **Manage stress**: Chronic stress can increase blood pressure, raise inflammation, and elevate cortisol levels, all of which are harmful to heart health. Finding ways to manage stress is essential. Practices such as mindfulness, meditation, deep breathing exercises, or simply spending time in nature can help reduce stress levels and support heart health.
- **Get quality sleep**: Sleep is essential for heart health, as it allows your body to repair and rejuvenate. Poor sleep can lead

to high blood pressure, increased inflammation, and a higher risk of heart disease. Aim for seven to nine hours of sleep each night, and practise good sleep hygiene by establishing a consistent bedtime routine and minimising screen time before sleep.
- **Avoid smoking and alcohol**: Smoking is one of the most significant risk factors for heart disease, as it damages blood vessels and increases the likelihood of plaque buildup. If you smoke, quitting is one of the best decisions you can make for your heart. Additionally, excessive alcohol consumption can raise blood pressure and contribute to weight gain. While drinking in moderation was once considered acceptable, the latest WHO guidelines state that no amount of alcohol is safe for the body.[10]
- **Maintain a healthy weight**: Being overweight or obese puts additional strain on your heart and increases the risk of developing heart disease. Achieving and maintaining a healthy weight through a combination of balanced eating and regular exercise can reduce these risks. Focus on making gradual, sustainable changes rather than resorting to crash diets.

Monitor Your Heart Health

You are making positive changes, but how can you be sure they are working? Visit your doctor yearly for blood pressure, cholesterol, and blood sugar tests. Additionally, ask about advanced markers like ApoB, which measures the particles that clog arteries, and hs-CRP, which indicates inflammation levels. These tests are especially useful for detecting risks early in individuals of South Asian descent.

Putting It into Practice

You do not have to overhaul your entire lifestyle overnight. The key to a heart-healthy life is consistency. Start by setting small, realistic goals and gradually build upon them.

Begin with a 10-minute walk after every meal or by cutting down on processed foods. As you make these small changes, you will begin to see the positive impact on your energy levels, mood, and overall health.

Track your progress, stay motivated, and celebrate every milestone along the way. Whether it is walking a little further, eating more vegetables, or finally quitting smoking, each small step brings you closer to a healthier heart. Over time, these habits will become second nature, and you will find that taking care of your heart becomes a way of life.

You've Got This

By combining exercise, a heart-healthy diet, and positive lifestyle choices, you can significantly lower your risk of heart disease and live a long, active life. The most important thing is to take action now, regardless of your age or current fitness level. Your heart is your lifeline, and caring for it today will benefit you in the years to come.

6

Is It Possible to Detox Your Liver?

As you scroll through Instagram reels, you will come across plenty of detox remedies – celery juice, three-day cleanses, turmeric shots, or magic teas. The pitch is that they will 'flush toxins', 'cleanse your liver', or 'reverse years of damage overnight'. It is a compelling pitch, except that it is mostly a myth.

Let us ask the real question: can you *actually* detox your liver?

Short answer: your liver does not need a fancy detox. It is the detox centre of the body.

Know Your Liver

Everyone knows what the heart and brain do, but the liver often gets overlooked. It is one of the hardest-working organs in your body, acting as a chemical processing plant that performs over 500 vital functions, detoxification being its most well-known role.

Everything you eat, drink, or inhale – whether it is alcohol, medications, pollutants, pesticides, hormones, or metabolic waste – gets broken down by the liver in a multi-phase process. These substances are converted into forms that can be safely eliminated either through the kidneys into the urine or through bile into the intestines.

Your liver does not store toxins like a dirty kitchen sponge. Instead, it is constantly processing and clearing them from the body.

The Real Liver Crisis

Here is where it gets serious: liver disease in India is not rare, and it is not just related to alcohol consumption.

Nearly 38 per cent of Indians are affected by non-alcoholic fatty liver disease (NAFLD).[11] Alarmingly, it is estimated that 35 per cent of Indian children have NAFLD. It is a silent epidemic. Most people do not even know they have it until it reaches an advanced stage. The good news is that NAFLD is reversible, especially when detected early. Correcting lifestyle factors can bring liver health back on track. That is why awareness is key.

So, Can You Detox Your Liver?

Not in the way you think, or influencers would like you to believe. You cannot magically 'flush' the liver. But you *can* support its detoxification functions by doing the following actions:

- **Eat for your liver**: Eat foods that support the liver's detoxification pathways. Include plenty of cruciferous vegetables (cauliflower, cabbage, radish, turnip, mustard greens), garlic, turmeric (in cooking, not as capsules), citrus fruits, and antioxidant-rich foods like amla, guava, and papaya. Cut back on sugar, refined carbs, and UPFs, all of which can increase fat accumulation in the liver.
- **Exercise regularly**: Aim for 150+ minutes of exercise each week. This translates to just 30 minutes, 5 days a week. This is the minimum amount of exercise anyone should strive for. Both strength-training and cardiovascular workouts help reduce fat accumulation in the liver and improve insulin sensitivity.
- **Sleep seven to eight hours per night**: Do not underestimate the power of sleep. Poor sleep can disrupt blood sugar levels and hormones, and increase inflammation, all of which can burden the liver.
- **Say NO to alcohol**: Everybody knows this, but we continue normalising alcohol in our everyday lives. If you care for your liver, alcohol needs to be shown the door immediately.
- **Hydrate smart**: No copper bottles or alkaline water nonsense. Just drink enough plain water throughout the day.
- **Do not poison your liver**: The market is flooded with herbal weight-loss supplements, alcohol-based 'tonics' masquerading as medicines, and supplements adulterated with heavy metals. Be wise and avoid these.
- **Stress less**: Chronic stress leads to chronic inflammation, overloading the liver. Try to set aside 10–15 minutes for activities like meditation, journalling, or pranayama, all of which are known to reduce stress levels.

These are boring, basic things that work – not karela shots or any other juice cleanses.

Air Pollution and Your Liver

Think pollution only affects your lungs? Think again. When you breathe in toxic air, microscopic particles enter your bloodstream and travel to the liver, increasing its detox workload. Chronic exposure to poor air has been linked to liver inflammation and even fatty liver disease, which is especially concerning in Indian cities with a high air quality index (AQI).

While moving to a cleaner-air location overnight is not feasible, there are steps you can take to protect yourself:
- Wear N95 masks on high AQI days.
- Maintain clean indoor air using ventilation and air purifiers.
- Support your liver with antioxidant-rich foods like amla, turmeric, berries, and green tea.
- Stay well-hydrated to help flush out toxins.

Living in India today means your liver has to work harder than ever. Give it the backup it needs.

Putting It into Practice

- Say no alcohol.
- Steer clear of herbal supplements or tonics.
- Include cruciferous vegetables in your everyday diet.
- Focus on exercise and sleep.

You've Got This

Your liver is a dynamic, intelligent organ that knows exactly what to do if you stop getting in its way. Instead of spending money on an expensive 'cleanse' twice a year, try adopting a lifestyle that supports your liver every single day. That is the true detox – and it costs way less.

7

Microbiome Matters: Decoding Gut Health

Social media is full of self-proclaimed 'gut health coaches' promising to fix everything from bloating to brain fog. The term 'gut health' has gained significant popularity in recent times, with Google searches increasing tenfold over the past five years. But what does it really mean, and why should you care?

In simple terms, gut health refers to how well your digestive system is functioning. A healthy gut efficiently processes food, absorbs nutrients, and keeps unwanted invaders in check, all while maintaining your overall health. However, dig a little deeper, and you will discover that gut health is about much more than just digestion. Your gut microbes have far-reaching effects on almost every aspect of your bodily functions.

The Gut Microbiome

Say hello to your gut microbiome – often referred to as your 'second brain'. It is packed with over 100 million neurons, home to 70 per cent of your immune system, and responsible for producing about 90 per cent of your body's serotonin. This bustling ecosystem of over 100 trillion microorganisms, which includes bacteria, fungi, and viruses, calls your digestive tract home and does far more than just hang around. These tiny tenants help digest food, regulate immune function, influence your metabolism and weight, and produce neurotransmitters like serotonin and dopamine that directly affect your mood and mental health. Emerging research suggests they may even influence long-term health and longevity.

A balanced gut microbiome (known as eubiosis) is diverse and stable, helping everything run smoothly. However, when the balance tips due to UPFs, chronic stress, or overuse of antibiotics, dysbiosis sets in. The result is inflammation, poor digestion, and an increased risk of metabolic disorders.

What You Eat Shapes Your Gut Microbiome

What you eat directly feeds your gut bacteria, influencing which strains thrive and which ones die. A diet rich in fibre, fermented foods, and whole, unprocessed ingredients promotes good bacteria. Meanwhile, UPFs – such as sugary snacks, refined grains, and artificial additives (most of which are mass-produced in factories) – fuel the growth of less beneficial microbes that make you crave the same junk food.

But there's good news. Your diet can nurture your gut microbiome and improve digestion, immunity, and even mental clarity. The key players here are probiotics and prebiotics.

Know Your Probiotics

Probiotic foods are all the rage. People are increasingly getting on the fermented foods bandwagon, either making them at home or buying commercially available options, like kombucha, yoghurt, kimchi, kefir, and so on.

Probiotic foods contain live, beneficial bacteria that support a healthy gut microbiome. They increase the number and diversity of gut bacteria, making digestion smoother and reducing inflammation. Various traditional fermented foods across cultures are naturally rich in probiotics, including:

- Indian-origin foods like homemade yoghurt (*dahi*), *kaanji*, fermented rice-based dishes (*pazhaiya sadam* and *pakhala*), and pickles.
- Probiotic foods from other parts of the world like kefir, kimchi, sauerkraut, miso, kombucha, lacto-fermented hot sauces, etc.

It is important to know that not all store-bought 'probiotic' foods contain live bacteria. Many mass-produced yoghurt drinks are high in sugar, and many packaged fermented foods are pasteurised to extend shelf life, which kills the beneficial bacteria in the process. When choosing a probiotic food, check the label and avoid products that contain added vinegar, excessive sugar, or artificial sweeteners. A long shelf life or expiry period could also indicate that the product has been pasteurised.

Consume probiotic-rich foods regularly, aiming for one serving per day. Keep varying the sources to get a variety of bacterial strains in your diet. Even though these bacterial strains are mostly resistant to stomach acids, having them as part of your meal buffers stomach acidity, enhancing the survival of these bacteria. While some bacteria will succumb to the stomach's acid, a significant portion will reach the intestines, especially when consumed alongside other foods.

Prebiotics: Gut Microbes' Favourite Food

I came across this line in a video, and it stayed with me: 'Do not be selfish and eat just for yourself. You also need to eat to feed the 100 trillion bacteria in your gut.' We are talking about prebiotics here.

If probiotics are the good bacteria, prebiotics are the fuel that keeps them thriving. Prebiotics are foods that contain a specific kind of dietary fibre, which remains undigested as it passes into the large intestine. There, it becomes food for the gut bacteria. These bacteria, in turn, produce short-chain fatty acids (SCFAs) that improve digestion, boost immunity, and enhance metabolic health.

Most prebiotics are your everyday foods that you can mindfully include in your diet without any additional shopping or effort. You do not need too much to keep your gut microbes well-fed and happy.

Here is a list of common prebiotic foods:
- Onion, garlic, bananas, raw bananas, apples, and flaxseeds
- Whole grains like oats, barley, and brown rice
- Chicory root (chicory powder is often added to ground coffee beans to make South Indian filter coffee)
- Polyphenols, which are colourful compounds found in plants like berries, dark chocolate (70 per cent or more cocoa), tea, coffee, nuts, seeds, and colourful veggies. These compounds act as antioxidants and also help nourish beneficial gut microbes.

To fuel these microbes effectively with diverse prebiotics and beneficial compounds, aim for variety in your plant intake. A great target is to try and consume 30 or more different types of plant foods each week. This includes all vegetables, fruits, whole grains, legumes (such as beans and lentils), nuts, seeds, and spices.

Beyond Diet

While food plays the main character in the movie titled 'Gut Microbiome', you will be surprised to know that lifestyle factors such as sleep, stress, exercise, and medication use also play critical roles. Without these factors, the narrative would be incomplete.

- **Stress and sleep**: Chronic stress and sleep deprivation can disrupt gut bacteria, leading to digestive issues. To combat this, try relaxation techniques like deep breathing, yoga, or a short daily walk.
- **Antibiotics**: While some bacterial infections may require your doctor to prescribe antibiotics, these medications wipe out both good and bad bacteria. If you have recently taken antibiotics, focus on eating probiotic- and prebiotic-rich foods to restore balance. Some antibiotic formulations even contain an extra dose of lactobacilli. Never take antibiotics without a prescription.
- **Other medications and chemicals**: If you are in the habit of popping a painkiller at the first sign of a headache, be aware that this can also damage the gut microbiome. It is good to limit the unnecessary use of painkillers, germicidal floor and kitchen cleaners in the house, and regular use of hand sanitisers to keep gut microbes happy.
- **Exercise**: Moderate exercise improves gut microbiome diversity and function, supporting digestion and overall health.

Putting It into Practice

Want to start improving your gut health today? Here are two easy steps to follow:
- Eat one probiotic and one prebiotic food daily. For example, begin your day with yoghurt and a banana, or add flaxseeds to your smoothie.
- Reduce your intake of UPFs. Each time you feel like reaching for a bag of chips or farsan, opt for a handful of roasted makhana, roasted chana, or nuts instead.

You've Got This

Think of your gut microbiome as a garden. Nurture it, and it will thrive. Small, mindful changes in your diet and lifestyle can transform your digestion and overall well-being. Keep in mind that you do not need fancy supplements, extreme diets, or a gut health coach – just focus on real, whole foods and maintain some consistency.

8

Activate Your Inner Calm: The Vagus Nerve Guide

At 60, Rajiv had accepted his constant bloating, poor sleep, and persistent stress as 'just age catching up'. But after watching an informative video about the vagus nerve and the benefits of activating it, he decided to try deep breathing exercises and humming (yes, you read that right). Over a few weeks, he noticed subtle but steady changes. His sleep became deeper, he felt calmer, and even his digestion improved. He was surprised that something so simple could make him feel so much better.

The Vagus Nerve

If you often feel anxious or on edge, in constant fight-or-flight mode, then you need to make the vagus nerve your new best friend. This nerve can help you chill out, sleep better, digest your food, and even regulate inflammation.

The vagus nerve is like a superhighway connecting the brain to key organs, including the gut, heart, lungs, liver, and pancreas. It plays a central role in regulating digestion, heart rate, respiratory function, and aspects of inflammation through the parasympathetic nervous system.

While the sympathetic system pumps you up to fight, fear, or flee, the parasympathetic system, with the vagus nerve as its most valuable player (MVP), brings you back to baseline. In a world full of alerts, stress, and chronic inflammation, learning to activate your vagus nerve is like hitting the reset button for your body and mind.

Why the Vagus Nerve Holds the Key to Your Calm

Chronic stress does not just make you feel frazzled; it increases cortisol, impairs digestion, disturbs sleep, affects immunity, and lays the foundation for lifestyle diseases. Your vagus nerve helps bring the body back into balance after stress by:
- Slowing the heart rate
- Promoting deep, relaxed breathing
- Improving digestion and gut motility
- Reducing systemic inflammation
- Enhancing mood through regulation of neurotransmitters (e.g., serotonin and gamma-aminobutyric acid [GABA])

A well-functioning vagus nerve means a better-regulated nervous system, which leads to more resilience, better sleep, calmer moods, and healthier digestion.

The Science Behind 'Vagal Tone'

Think of vagal tone as your nervous system's fitness level. A higher vagal tone means that your body can recover quickly from stress and regulate itself more efficiently.

Researchers often measure this through HRV, which can now be tracked with some wearable devices, like the Apple Watch. HRV refers to the variation in time between your heartbeats. A higher HRV reflects better vagal activity and is associated with lower inflammation, improved mood, and reduced risk of chronic disease.

The good news is that vagal tone is trainable. Anyone can naturally stimulate the vagus nerve through simple daily practices, without needing any fancy gadgets.

Your Toolkit to Stimulate the Vagus Nerve

- **Slow, deep breathing**: Breathe in for four counts and breathe out for six to eight counts. This long exhale triggers the vagus nerve and shifts your body into relaxation mode. Just five minutes a day of this can make a noticeable difference.
- **Humming, chanting, or singing**: The vagus nerve is connected to your vocal cords. Humming with lips closed,

chanting 'om', singing, or even gargling can stimulate this nerve. In fact, singing with others also releases oxytocin, the bonding hormone.
- **Cold exposure**: Splashing your face with cold water, dipping your face into a bowl of cold water for 30 seconds, or taking a brief cold shower can activate the vagus nerve through the body's natural diving reflex. This slows down your heart rate and signals your nervous system to shift to a more relaxed state.
- **Meditation and mindfulness**: Practices such as loving-kindness meditation and body scan practices have been shown to boost vagal tone. Several videos on YouTube offer these kinds of guided meditations. Regular practice improves emotional regulation and HRV.
- **Gut health support**: Since the vagus nerve directly connects the brain and gut, keeping your microbiome healthy with fibre, prebiotics, and fermented foods enhances communication in both directions.
- **Social connection and laughter**: Genuine connection stimulates the vagus nerve and calms the body. This is why hugging someone you trust feels so good. Now you know that the senior citizens' laughter clubs in your neighbourhood parks are no laughing matter.
- **Yoga**: Certain yoga practices, especially those that incorporate breathwork, chanting, and gentle movement, are powerful vagus stimulators.

Putting It into Practice

- A 10-minute evening wind-down ritual that includes three minutes of chanting 'om' or humming, five minutes of slow breathing (inhale for four seconds and exhale for six seconds), and two minutes of gratitude journalling can help lower your heart rate, shift you into parasympathetic mode, and improve your sleep quality.
- Feeling anxious or overwhelmed during the day? Splash cold water on your face 10 to 15 times, or dip your face into a bowl of iced water. This can stimulate the vagus nerve and provide a quick reset for your nervous system.

You've Got This

You do not need to meditate for hours or follow a rigid wellness routine to stimulate your vagus nerve. Small, consistent habits like humming, laughing with friends, or practising slow breathing before bedtime are powerful ways to bring your body back to a state of calm.

In a world that constantly pushes us into overdrive, the vagus nerve acts as your built-in brake system. Learn to use it, and you will find it easier to navigate stress and support your long-term health from the inside out.

9

The Great Energy Heist

Do you remember that boundless energy of your youth that you often took for granted? When you could power through the day, chase your dreams, cook dinner, call a friend, even dance late into the night without needing a nap or caffeine? That seemingly infinite energy was your baseline. But somewhere along the way, that changed.

Energy is what powers everything meaningful in life: caring for yourself and others, eating well, exercising, connecting with people, and contributing to the world. As we age, energy becomes something we cannot afford to take for granted. It is not just about 'keeping up'; it is about reclaiming the vitality that lets us fully engage with life.

If you wake up feeling tired, need multiple cups of coffee just to function, or find yourself skipping the gym because you are already exhausted, it is your body asking for a different kind of fuel.

Here is the good news: energy is not just a relic of your 20s. It is renewable, and it comes in two forms:
- **Physical energy**, which powers your body
- **Mental energy**, which fuels your focus and emotional stamina

Let us break it down further.

Physical Energy

Food: Fuelling your body with the right nutrition

Let's take the simple example of a car. If the fuel tank is empty, the car will not move. If you fill its tank with cheap, low-quality fuel, its performance suffers. Similarly, food is our fuel, and getting the right nutrients is essential for maintaining energy levels. Deficiencies in key vitamins and minerals are some of the biggest culprits behind constant fatigue.

- **Iron**: If you experience sluggishness or breathlessness after minimal activity or frequent headaches, low iron may be the reason. This mineral is crucial for transporting oxygen in the blood; without it, your cells cannot obtain the energy they need. Women, in particular, are more prone to iron deficiency due to menstruation, especially if they have heavy periods.
- **Vitamin D**: Many people living in urban India today seem to be deficient in vitamin D. This fat-soluble vitamin plays a vital role in muscle strength and immune function. A deficiency can leave you feeling weak and perpetually tired.
- **Vitamin B12**: Essential for brain function and nerve health, a lack of vitamin B12 can lead to fatigue, memory issues, and mood imbalances.
- **Magnesium**: Often known as the 'relaxation mineral', magnesium helps with muscle function and sleep. Deficiencies can contribute to stress, muscle cramps, and low energy.

A well-fed body runs on real food, not pills. While supplements can fill genuine gaps, such as vitamins D or B12, they are no substitute for a diverse, whole-food diet. When in doubt, do not guess; get your blood tests done.

Movement: Energy creates energy

It may sound counterintuitive, but the more you move, the more energy you generate. Regular exercise boosts circulation, improves oxygen delivery, and increases the release of endorphins – all things that leave you feeling more alive.

- Strength training preserves muscle mass, which naturally declines with age, making us feel weaker and more fatigued.
- Cardio exercises, such as walking, swimming, HIIT, or cycling, improve heart health and oxygenation, keeping us energised throughout the day.
- Stretching and mobility exercises ensure that stiffness and discomfort do not drain your energy before you even get started.

Do note that over-exercising, especially without proper recovery, can lead to burnout and fatigue. Always listen to your body.

Sleep: The most overlooked energy booster

Many people look for external solutions to their low energy, such as supplements, special diets, or energy drinks, while completely missing the most powerful tool of all – sleep.

Poor sleep disrupts everything from hormone balance to cognitive function. Here is how to optimise it:
- Prioritise deep sleep by keeping your bedroom cool, dark, and screen-free before bedtime.
- Follow a consistent schedule. Your body thrives on routine.
- Avoid stimulants late in the day, like caffeine and heavy meals.
- Drink most of your water for the day well before bedtime to prevent being woken up in the middle of the night by a full bladder.

The quality of sleep is more important than the duration. Eight hours of interrupted sleep is not as restorative as six hours of deep, uninterrupted rest.

Mental Energy

Feeling physically fine but mentally exhausted? Mental energy is all about focus. And where your attention goes, your energy flows.

Prevent energy leaks

Ever wondered why scrolling social media for an hour leaves you feeling drained? This happens because your brain is burning energy like the central processor of a computer, processing an endless stream of information, most of which is useless.
- Set boundaries with social media and news consumption. While the constant stimulation may seem entertaining or productive, it is extremely draining.
- The same applies to unproductive conversations, such as gossip, negativity, or arguments.
- Say no freely. Be selective about commitments; otherwise, you will end up spreading yourself too thin.

Manage stress before it becomes your manager

Chronic stress is one of the biggest drains on mental energy. When your brain is constantly in fight-or-flight mode, it is consuming resources at an unsustainable rate.
- Practise mindfulness or meditation. Even five minutes of deep breathing with long exhalations can reset your nervous system.
- Schedule intentional breaks. Taking short breaks to step away from work for a walk or stretch can boost mental clarity.
- Prioritise joy. Hobbies, laughter, and playtime with loved ones or pets recharge your mental battery.
- Spend time in nature. Go for walks in parks, take a stroll down a tree-lined street, or even around your building if you do not have access to parks, and leave your phone at home whenever possible.

Purpose fuels energy

Ever notice how you can spend hours doing something you love and not feel drained? That is because passion generates energy. When you engage in meaningful work, whether creative, social, or intellectual, your mental energy expands rather than depletes.

If you constantly feel drained, ask yourself if you are spending energy on things that matter to you. If not, it is time to reassess where you place your focus.

The Physical and Mental Energy Connection

Physical and mental energy do not exist in silos; they feed off each other. A poor diet leads to brain fog. Lack of movement makes you feel sluggish. Stress and anxiety cause physical exhaustion. The key to sustained energy is balancing both aspects. With some simple practices, you can become a pro at it.

Putting It into Practice

- Eat nutritious food so your brain and body function optimally.
- Move your body so you feel more alive and less stuck.
- Sleep deeply to restore your reserves.
- Set boundaries on mental clutter to protect your focus.
- Do things that bring you joy and purpose to create energy rather than just consume it.

You've Got This

Start by addressing any one area of your lifestyle that feels the most depleted, whether it is nutrition, sleep, movement, or mental clarity. Small, consistent changes will build over time, giving you the energy you need to live a full, vibrant life. Because, at the end of the day, having energy means having the capacity to live life to the fullest.

10

Making Fat Loss Happen: A Real-World Manual

This could well be the world's most asked question: How do I lose fat? It's what drives people to spend billions chasing answers through fat-burning teas, crash diets, and the latest wearables. But is there really a hidden secret known only to a chosen few? Or have we simply been looking in the wrong places all along?

Fat loss is not magic; it is all about metabolism. And metabolism follows science, not fads. If you understand how your body stores and burns fat, you can stop chasing shortcuts and start making real progress, steadily and sustainably.

Let us break down what actually needs to happen for fat loss to kick in and remain consistent.

Why Does Your Body Love to Store Fat?

Our bodies are still coded for the Stone Age. Back then, food was scarce. Famine, drought, and migration were real threats. As a result, the body evolved to store excess energy as fat, which is a compact and long-lasting fuel reserve. One gram of fat holds over twice the energy of carbs or protein, making it perfect for survival. Fat was our biological power bank: slow to charge, but reliable in tough times.

When you eat more calories than your body needs, that extra energy is stored for later, mostly in the form of triglycerides inside fat cells (adipocytes). These fat cells can be called upon during times of fasting, exertion, or food scarcity.

Today, while the code remains the same, the world has changed. We are surrounded by food and 10-minute deliveries. We move less;

we stress over emails, not predators. We are wired for famine while sitting in front of an endless buffet. Think of it as using a pager in the era of smartphones. It made sense then, but not now. Except we cannot upgrade our body's operating system.

That is why understanding fat loss through the lens of evolution is key. When you align with your biology, you stop fighting your body and start working with it.

To Lose Fat, You Need a Sustained Energy Deficit

Fat loss happens when your body needs more energy than it can get from food. In this state, it turns to its stored energy reserves, with fat being the largest source. That's the golden rule: you will lose fat when there is a shortage of energy. This condition is known as a calorie deficit, which can be achieved in several ways:
- Consuming fewer calories
- Increasing calorie expenditure through physical activity
- A combination of both: eating fewer calories and increasing physical activity (the most effective strategy)

The body does not burn fat just because you did a 'fat-burning workout' or ate a particular type of food. It burns fat when it needs to make up for an energy shortfall.

What Happens to Fat During Weight Loss?

Here is where it gets fascinating. Fat does not get 'burnt off' like a piece of firewood; instead, it is metabolised. Triglycerides stored in fat cells are broken down into fatty acids and glycerol. These are released into the bloodstream and transported to the liver and muscles, where they are converted into ATP (energy), carbon dioxide, and water.

The carbon dioxide produced is exhaled through the lungs, while the water is lost via urine, sweat, and breath. So, you literally breathe out fat. Roughly 84 per cent of fat is exhaled as carbon dioxide, and the remaining 16 per cent is lost as water. Fat does not 'melt' or 'get flushed out'; it gets oxidised (broken down using oxygen) and exits your body through your breath and body fluids.

What Makes Fat Loss Stall or Slow Down?

The body does not like to be in an energy deficit for too long. It adapts. Some common metabolic adaptations and errors that can stall fat loss include the following:

- Reduced NEAT (non-exercise activity thermogenesis) – you unconsciously move less
- Underestimating calorie intake – even healthy food can be overeaten
- Overestimating exercise burn
- Loss of muscle mass from extreme dieting – lowers your resting metabolic rate
- Hormonal changes – such as perimenopause, stress (cortisol), or poor thyroid function

These factors do not 'break' your metabolism, but they can slow things down. Adjusting your strategy, being consistent, and staying calm are key to overcoming these challenges.

All Weight Loss Is Not Fat Loss

Fat loss means reducing body fat percentage. Weight loss can also include the following:

- Water loss (especially when carbs are reduced)
- Muscle loss (if protein is low or strength training is missing)
- Digestive residue or food weight

This is why obsessing over the scale can mislead and demotivate. Use multiple markers like how your clothes fit, measurements, photos, strength gains, and your overall sense of well-being.

Science-Backed Ways to Achieve Fat Loss

- **Maintain a slight but consistent calorie deficit**: Do not starve. Aim to eat just enough below your maintenance needs (usually 300–500 kcal daily) to make it sustainable.
- **Increase protein intake**: This supports muscle retention, satiety, and thermogenesis (your body burns more calories processing protein).
- **Incorporate strength training**: Strength training is the best way to preserve muscle mass and keep metabolism humming.

Cardio supports heart health and calorie burn, but resistance training is a must for long-term fat loss.
- **Prioritise good sleep and stress management**: High levels of stress and poor sleep can lead to elevated cortisol, poor insulin sensitivity, increased cravings, and fat retention.
- **Stay hydrated and practise deep breathing**: Water supports fat metabolism and helps with fat loss by enabling fat oxidation. Deep, relaxed breathing (like during pranayama or walking) ensures optimal oxygenation, supporting the breakdown of fat into carbon dioxide and water.
- **Commit to consistency and patience**: No 'seven-day fat burn' is going to give you lasting results. Aim for 0.5–1 kg of fat loss per week. It may feel slow – but over months, it adds up to big changes.

Putting It into Practice

- Start tracking your intake for three to five days, just to see where you are.
- Include a strength workout two to three times per week and aim for 7,000–10,000 steps a day.
- Add 10–15 g more protein per day and drink an extra two to three glasses of water.

You've Got This

Fat loss does not mean fighting your body. When you combine knowledge with consistency, change is inevitable. You do not need extreme discipline; you need an approach you can stick to, and fat loss will happen.

11

Fad-Proof Your Health

The modern health scene feels like a whirlwind, with new fads every week, gadgets that claim to monitor every physiological metric, miracle cures, and an overwhelming flood of information. It is easy to get swept up in all of it, especially when the advice comes from seemingly knowledgeable voices on podcasts, YouTube channels, and social media followings in the millions. That is the power of numbers. However, true health advice must be rooted in solid science rather than the fleeting claims of viral influencers.

The Four Pillars

Before you try the latest trend, take a moment to pause. Are your health foundations in place? Chasing trends without addressing the basics is like decorating a house without building the structure first. The four non-negotiable pillars of health are as follows:
- Balanced nutrition
- Regular physical activity
- Quality sleep
- Stress management

If you have got these dialled in, you are already doing the heavy lifting. No supplement, biohacking gadget, or detox tea can replace these basics. Yet, trends often lure us in because they seem exciting and easier. Quick fixes always sound more appealing than long-term habits. But most trends do not last. Some are harmless but ineffective; others can be downright dangerous.

So, how do you tell what is worth trying and what is simply another fad? Let us break it down.

The Health Trend Lifecycle

Every few months, a new health craze takes over social media, promising extraordinary results. If you regularly use X (formerly Twitter), you will find many accounts run by people I like to call 'health bros' posting lengthy threads about their latest experiment, all based solely on personal experience. These anecdotes quickly turn into gospel without a shred of scientific evidence backing them.

We have all heard of various trends, such as juice cleanses, raw food diets, carnivore eating, extreme fasting, and ice baths. Some, like intermittent fasting, gain scientific credibility and become part of mainstream health advice, while others lose popularity as research exposes them as ineffective or even risky.

Why do these trends thrive? It's a combination of slick marketing, wellness influencers, and the powerful psychology of hope. Social media is flooded with aspirational morning routines, supplement stacks, and diet hacks. However, real health is not built on what is trending but on what is true.

How to Evaluate a Health Trend – What Is Worth It?

Before jumping on the next big thing, ask yourself these questions, or what I like to call a Trend Evaluation Checklist:

- Is it science-backed? Look for high-quality studies rather than just personal stories. Evidence-based medicine (SORT A-level) should be the gold standard, which anyone can fact-check today on ChatGPT.
- Is it sustainable? Can you realistically follow this for months or years? If not, it is likely just a short-term fix.
- Who does it benefit? Not all trends are one-size-fits-all. For example, while intermittent fasting may help metabolic health, it can disrupt hormonal balance in some women.
- Does it carry risks? Could it worsen an existing condition? Keto, for instance, can elevate cholesterol levels, and raw diets can cause digestive distress.

This simple checklist can help you separate what is helpful from what is hype and tailor trends to your personal health needs.

A Closer Look at Some Popular Health Trends

- **Intermittent fasting**: Backed by solid evidence for metabolic health and longevity. But it can be problematic for those with hormonal imbalances or eating disorders.
- **Cold plunges and saunas**: There are proven benefits associated with improved circulation, stress resilience, and muscle recovery. Nevertheless, extreme temperature shifts can be life-threatening.
- **Keto and carnivore diets**: These diets can be effective for fast weight loss and metabolic health but are difficult to sustain and may have long-term implications for cardiovascular health.
- **Detoxes and juice cleanses**: The word 'detox' is a marketing gimmick. Your liver and kidneys already perform detoxification perfectly well.
- **Personalised supplements and biohacking**: These approaches are intriguing, and in some cases promising, but still experimental, costly, and not always evidence-backed.

What works for one person may not work for another. Personalisation, sustainability, and safety are the keys.

The Hidden Dangers of Chasing Health Trends

You might wonder, what's the harm in experimenting? But the risks are real:

- **Financial cost**: Expensive supplements, gadgets, and diets can burn a hole in your wallet with little to show for it.
- **Delaying actual treatment**: It may prevent or delay you from taking the proper treatment for your condition, such as people trying out alternative medicine modalities for cancer.
- **Worsening health**: Juice cleanses can destabilise blood sugar in diabetics. Extreme fasting can disrupt hormonal balance in women. Unregulated supplement use can be dangerous.
- **Mental health toll**: Constantly chasing the 'next best thing' can create stress and obsession.

Putting It into Practice

- Question everything. If it sounds too good to be true, it probably is.

- Seek reputable sources. Rely on information from established medical organisations, peer-reviewed journals, and licensed healthcare professionals, not Instagram reels.
- Consult your doctor. Always discuss any new health trends or treatments with your physician, not your favourite influencer, before trying them.
- Prioritise evidence-based medicine. Focus on treatments and practices that are supported by scientific evidence.

You've Got This

Health choices should be grounded in science and personalised to your body, not based on social media buzz or someone else's biohacking experiment. Stay open-minded, but do not lose sight of the fundamentals. Because when you focus on the four foundational pillars, you will rarely go wrong.

12
Health Check-Ups: Your Annual Power Move

Good health is not always predictable, and a health issue can catch people off guard. But we do not have to accept this unpredictability passively.

Good businesses invest in trend analysis and company health reports. It is only sensible for us to invest in our own body's health trends and reports, helping us make informed decisions before problems escalate. That is exactly what regular health check-ups offer: a proactive strategy rather than a reactive response.

People often wait for symptoms to appear before visiting a doctor. But conditions like high blood sugar, thyroid imbalances, hypertension, or even cancer can develop silently. The purpose of routine screenings is not to chase numbers; it is to identify patterns early, before a disease sends its roots deep into your body.

This chapter will help you understand which tests truly matter, how to personalise your check-ups, and what to do with the results. By doing so, you can use this powerful tool for lifelong wellness.

Investment, Not Expense

Think of your annual health check-up as your body's financial audit. These screenings allow you to track your metabolic, hormonal, and cardiovascular health before minor imbalances snowball into something catastrophic or a chronic condition.

For example, prediabetes caught early is often reversible. But undiagnosed high blood sugar can silently damage blood vessels, raising your risk of heart disease and nerve damage. Similarly, identifying high levels of LDL cholesterol or elevated inflammatory markers early gives you the chance to address them through lifestyle changes before medication becomes mandatory.

Regular check-ups can reduce long-term healthcare costs, hospitalisations, and the risk of disease progression. In short, what you spend today may save you years of medical bills, discomfort, and irreversible damage.

Your Smart Health Check-Up Strategy

The challenge with annual check-ups is that not all tests are necessary for everyone. The healthcare industry often promotes generic, one-size-fits-all packages, at most giving different packages for men and women and a few variations for different age groups. What you truly need depends on several factors:
- Your age and gender
- Family history: a parent with diabetes, heart disease, or autoimmune conditions may make those your priority tests
- Lifestyle and risk factors: smoking, sedentary living, and chronic stress raise your cardiovascular risk
- Existing health conditions, like thyroid issues, PCOS, or metabolic syndrome, which require more targeted and frequent monitoring

Essential Tests by Life Stage

In your 20s and 30s: Laying the foundation
- **Annual**: Blood pressure, fasting blood sugar, thyroid panel (TSH, T3, T4), complete blood count (CBC), vitamin D, and vitamin B12
- **Every two to three years**: Lipid profile, liver and kidney function tests, iron studies, Pap smear (women), testicular exam (men)
- **Lifestyle-based**: Gut microbiome testing (for chronic bloating or IBS), advanced metabolic panels (if insulin resistance is suspected)

In your 40s: Proactive disease prevention

Everything above, plus:
- **Every one to two years**: ECG or stress test (for heart health), mammogram (women), prostate screening (men)

- **Optional**: Continuous glucose monitoring (CGM) for metabolic trends (especially if diabetic), DEXA scan for body composition

In your 50s and beyond: Longevity and functional health

All of the above, plus:
- Bone density test (osteoporosis risk)
- Hearing and vision screening
- Regular inflammation markers (hs-CRP, homocysteine) for cardiovascular health

Metabolic health is increasingly recognised as a key marker of longevity. Tests like fasting insulin and CGM data (even in non-diabetics) can reveal dysfunction years before a diagnosis is made.

Beyond Standard Tests: The Future of Personalised Preventive Health

In the last decade, health tracking has become more precise than ever. Consider integrating:
- **Gut microbiome testing**: Helps tailor diet, reduce inflammation, and optimise digestion
- **Genetic risk screening**: Identifies predispositions for diseases like Alzheimer's, heart disease, and certain cancers
- **Wearable tech**: Devices like Oura Rings, Apple Watches, and Whoop bands track HRV, sleep cycles, and stress adaptation

While not necessary for everyone, these innovations are making precision health more accessible.

Interpreting Your Results

Many people receive a health report and either panic or ignore it. Here is how to approach your results effectively.

Look at trends, not just one-time numbers. A slightly high cholesterol reading means little if your inflammation markers are low and overall heart health is strong.

Ask the right questions, including:
- Is this a temporary fluctuation or a true concern?
- What lifestyle shifts can improve this parameter?

- Do I need medication, or is there room to manage this naturally?

Avoid over-testing. Some results may lead to unnecessary worry or interventions. Have an open conversation with your doctor before reacting to borderline findings.

Prevention is powerful. Smart health check-ups offer clarity and course correction long before disease sets in.

Putting It into Practice

- Do not just get the tests done, but also understand them by consulting a doctor.
- Track key markers over time.
- Use insights to shape a stronger health strategy.

You've Got This

By shifting from reactive to proactive healthcare, you will ensure that your future self has better energy, resilience, and longevity.

13

Genetic Testing: The Truth Behind the Trend

Imagine having a manual for your body that tells you exactly which foods are good for you, how well you can tolerate caffeine or alcohol, what your risk is for certain health conditions, and so on. This may sound futuristic, but the future is already at our doorstep. It is called genetic testing.

Over the last few years, we have noticed a boom in at-home DNA tests that promise reports claiming to unlock the secrets of your body. However, can this tiny collection of saliva in a tube really provide you with life-changing insights? Genetic testing is not a fortune-telling crystal ball, but more like a torchlight in the dark, helping you gain awareness of clues about your body.

Let us explore the various genetic tests available presently, what they can reveal, and whether they are worth the cost.

The Types of Genetic Testing

Genetic testing broadly falls into four categories: carrier testing, prenatal, newborn, and predictive.

My first encounter with genetic testing occurred during medical college, where it was used in prenatal screening. Ultrasounds and blood tests helped detect abnormalities early in pregnancy. For high-risk pregnancies, more advanced tests like amniocentesis and chorionic villus sampling (CVS) were employed. Today, with IVF (in vitro fertilisation), the field has advanced even further. Preimplantation genetic testing allows embryos to be screened for chromosomal issues before implantation, increasing the chances of a healthy pregnancy. For monogenic diseases like thalassemia, where both partners are carriers, embryos can be screened to ensure that one with thalassemia major is not implanted.

Somewhere around 2010–2015, a turning point occurred when companies like 23andMe and AncestryDNA began offering direct-to-consumer DNA tests for tracing genealogy, capitalising on growing curiosity about personal heritage.

Predictive Genetic Testing

This chapter focuses primarily on predictive testing and whether it can support better ageing and longevity. These tests can reveal your genetic predisposition to conditions such as Alzheimer's, heart disease, breast cancer, and type 2 diabetes.

Your genetic makeup offers valuable insights into your future health and can help you make more informed decisions. When used well, this information supports preventive care and early intervention.

Unlike diagnostic tests that detect diseases already present, predictive tests estimate your risk of developing certain conditions. They analyse specific gene variations associated with increased susceptibility. Importantly, a positive result does not mean you *will* get the disease; it simply indicates a higher-than-average risk.

Most reputable centres offering genetic testing include pre- and post-test counselling. Pre-counselling helps you understand which tests are relevant for you, while post-counselling interprets results and translates them into actionable advice.

Dr Naresh Trehan, managing director of Medanta Hospitals, has highlighted the role of genetic testing in preventing heart attacks in young people. In an interview, he emphasised the value of early check-ups and genetic awareness: 'We know that for cardiac disease, gene detection is available. So if you know your propensity, you will be more careful about avoiding things that contribute to heart disease.'[12]

Key Predictive Tests Available in India

- **Breast and Ovarian Cancer (BRCA1/BRCA2)**: BRCA1 and BRCA2 genes, when mutated, significantly increase breast and ovarian cancer risk. The cost ranges from ₹4,000 to ₹25,000,

depending on the lab and type of test. The test requires blood or saliva samples.
- **Heart health**: Genetic markers can indicate a predisposition to inherited cholesterol disorders, which may increase the risk of heart disease. The cost ranges from ₹3,000 to ₹15,000, and the test requires blood samples.
- **Diabetes predisposition**: Genetic factors contribute to type 2 diabetes risk alongside lifestyle factors. The cost ranges from ₹2,500 to ₹10,000. Testing requires blood samples.
- While cancer, heart disease, and diabetes are often the most common health concerns, genetic testing also offers insights into neurological conditions like Alzheimer's disease (by checking for gene variations like the APOE-e4 allele).

While these tests offer valuable information, they do not offer certainty. They can only indicate the likelihood of developing a condition. Even if a test shows a higher risk of heart disease, diabetes, or cancer, it does not mean you will necessarily develop the disease.

So here is the question: does knowing your genetic risk change what you need to do?

If the solution still involves eating well, staying active, managing stress, and getting enough sleep, does the test justify the cost and the anxiety that follows?

Most preventive steps are the same whether or not you have taken a genetic test. In that sense, genetic testing does not replace the need for a healthy lifestyle. What it can do, however, is *motivate* someone to take action sooner or tailor their focus, especially if the risk is high or family history is significant.

On the other hand, the stress of knowing you carry a high-risk gene may outweigh the benefits, particularly if it leads to overthinking, fear-based choices, or unnecessary treatments.

The goal, then, should be to build a preventive mindset, regardless of whether you test your genes. Think of genetic testing as one more tool, not the entire toolbox. It can help in specific cases, such as when there is a strong family history of a disease or when making high-stakes reproductive decisions. But for the average person, it should not replace the fundamentals of good health: balanced food, physical activity, adequate rest, and regular medical care.

You've Got This

A genetic test is not mandatory to start making positive changes in your life. Move your body. Feed it what it actually recognises as food. Rest well. Reduce toxic exposures whenever possible. And if you do decide to take a gene test, do not let the results define you. Let them inform you, maybe even motivate you, but not intimidate you.

Part II

Food, Fad, and Fiction

1. When Guesswork Fails, Try Tracking
2. 'Eight Glasses a Day' and Other Hydration Myths
3. Balancing Blood Sugar Throughout the Day
4. Protein Panic: How Much Do You Need?
5. Whey Protein: Facts Over Fear
6. Fibre: The Unsung Hero of Your Diet (and Gut)
7. The Deficiency Myth: What Vegetarians Really Lack (and Don't)
8. Intermittent Fasting: What the Science Actually Says
9. Minimalist Eating: Why Variety Is Not Always the Spice of Life
10. Sugar: Friend, Foe, or Frenemy?
11. Fruit Fearmongering: A Wellness Trend Gone Wrong
12. The 'Gluten-Free' Lie
13. Which Cooking Oil Is Best for Your Health?
14. Is Organic Food Just a Fancy Label or a Smarter Choice?
15. The Whole Truth About Ultra-Processed Foods
16. Reading Nutrition Labels: The Truth Behind the Packaging
17. The Best Cooking Methods for Everyday Meals
18. The Iron-Strong Plate: A Food-First Strategy for Anaemia
19. Alcohol: What Are You Really Toasting?
20. Why We Eat When We Are Not Hungry

1

When Guesswork Fails, Try Tracking

Just eat healthy and exercise more; you do not need to count calories – that sounds comforting, doesn't it? It feels like advice from someone who genuinely cares. However, for many people balancing long work hours, family responsibilities, missed workouts, and the hormonal ups and downs of life, this advice can be as helpful as telling someone to 'just save more' when they are overwhelmed by bills. Such advice often leads to vague or no results at all.

This is where calorie tracking can be an incredibly effective ally. Rather than being a burden or obsession, it serves as a practical tool to help us understand and manage our energy intake, especially when we have specific health or fitness goals in mind.

Let us start with the basics.

Calories: The Currency of Energy

Calories are a unit of energy, and your body requires energy to function. Everything from your heartbeat to your morning walk, including brain activity and digesting food, uses calories. Here is where those calories typically go:

- **Basal metabolic rate (BMR)**: Roughly 60–75 per cent of your daily calorie expenditure occurs even while you are at rest. This process supports essential functions such as maintaining your heart rate, enabling your lungs to breathe, and regulating your body temperature.
- **Thermic effect of food (TEF)**: About 10 per cent of your caloric burn is used to digest and absorb the food you eat.
- **Physical activity**: The remaining 15–30 per cent of your calorie usage depends on your level of movement, including activities such as steps, workouts, and even fidgeting.

When you combine all of these factors, you arrive at your total daily energy expenditure (TDEE). This number represents the calories you need to consume in a day to maintain your current weight.

If your goal is to lose weight, you will need to create a calorie deficit by taking in slightly fewer calories than you burn.

Enter: Calorie Tracking

Calorie tracking transforms vague hunches into concrete data. It creates awareness about the food you eat.

Many of us believe we are eating 'just a little bit' of this or that: a few spoonfuls of rice while cooking, a handful of cashews while scrolling, or the leftover idli that no one touched. But those small bites could be slowly adding to your weight over the years.

Logging your meals, even for just a couple of weeks, offers clarity. You will start noticing patterns, such as what fills you up, what leaves you feeling hungry, and where those sneaky extras are creeping in. It becomes less about restriction and more about informed decision-making.

The Tech Makes It Easier

Gone are the days of scribbling in food diaries and flipping through calorie charts. Apps like MyFitnessPal, HealthifyMe, Cronometer, and Lose It! have made tracking much easier. Many of these apps now include Indian foods, barcode scanners, and saved meals for quick, one-click entries.

Some even have built-in AI that can estimate calorie content from food photos. Take a picture of your lunch, and you will get an estimate. While it may not be perfect, especially for complex dishes, it provides a helpful starting point, particularly if you find manual tracking tedious.

Beyond Numbers: What You Really Learn

Calorie tracking helps you understand your macronutrient balance beyond just counting calories. You notice details like:
- Are you eating enough protein?
- Are your meals overloaded with refined carbs?
- Is a significant portion of your fat intake coming from snacks?
- Are you missing out on fibre, the unsung hero of gut health?

You also learn which meals keep you full and energised, and which ones leave you craving sugar an hour later. Over time, many people find that they do not need to log their food daily. Instead, just a few 'reset' days per month are enough to stay on track.

But What About Accuracy?

There is a margin of error in nutrition labels, which can vary by up to 20 per cent. Additionally, entries for Indian food can vary significantly. Homemade dishes may have unpredictable amounts of oil, and even the same dish made by you or your cook can differ by as much as 200 calories. Furthermore, not all calories are absorbed in the same way; for example, whole almonds release less energy than almond butter.

However, having imperfect data is still better than having no data at all, as it can provide valuable insights.

If you enjoy working with data, you will likely find tracking enjoyable. If you dislike data, consider it a training tool to help you find balance.

When You Should Not Track

A note of caution: if you have struggled with disordered eating in the past, calorie tracking may feel triggering or obsessive. In such cases, it is better to work with a nutritionist or therapist.

Alternatives to Calorie Counting

- Focus on eating wholesome meals that include protein, healthy fats, and complex carbohydrates. It is much harder to binge on home-cooked rajma chawal than on chips.
- Aim for 1–1.5 g of protein per kg of body weight. Protein helps you feel full, maintains muscle, boosts TEF, stabilises blood sugar, and reduces cravings.
- Add a cup of non-starchy veggies to each meal. This single habit boosts fibre intake, provides essential micronutrients, and enhances satiety, while lowering calorie density.
- Listen to your body. Follow methods like intuitive eating, which involves recognising your body's hunger and fullness cues. This approach promotes a healthier long-term relationship with food. Remember that there are considerations beyond just calories and food. Factors like getting sufficient sleep, avoiding

extreme cardio (which can make you hungrier and lead to loss of muscle mass), and managing stress are all crucial for effective weight management. Depriving oneself and engaging in yo-yo dieting can be counterproductive.
- You do not need to count calories to know that meals from restaurants or takeaways are typically two to three times more calorie-dense than home-cooked meals. Eating out regularly is one of the quickest ways to gain weight, so try to make home-cooked meals the norm and reserve eating out as an occasional indulgence.

Putting It into Practice

Consider using a calorie-tracking app to identify your eating patterns. Log your meals honestly and notice patterns like high-calorie snacks or under-eating during main meals.

You've Got This

Calorie tracking is like using Google Maps for your meals. While you may eventually reach your destination without it, having a clear understanding of where you are starting, where you are headed, and the fastest route to get there can be incredibly beneficial. It is a smart tool when used with perspective and balance.

Just as your phone can tell you how many steps you took today or how long you slept the previous night, why not let it help you make better food choices as well?

2

'Eight Glasses a Day' and Other Hydration Myths

Feeling thirsty? Drink water. You would think that would be one of the simplest things in life, but sadly, it is not.

Social media has done its fair bit to stir up confusion around how to drink water correctly.

What type of water is best – alkaline, mineral, reverse osmosis, or distilled? What is the ideal temperature – warm, cold, or room temperature? Should you sit or stand while drinking?

Is it better to use a copper bottle, a steel bottle, or drink straight from a clay pot? And, of course, there is the big question of how much water you should drink: eight glasses, three to four litres, or a glass every hour?

Hydration, once an instinctive and straightforward act, has now been overcomplicated by misinformation, marketing, and half-baked wellness advice.

Let us bring the clarity back. Here is what science actually says regarding proper hydration.

Hydration Is Not a Number Game

The origins of the advice to drink 'eight glasses a day' are surprisingly misunderstood. In 1945, the US National Research Council recommended a daily water intake of approximately 2.5 litres for adults. However, it clearly noted that a significant portion of this requirement is naturally met through prepared foods, a detail that is often overlooked.

Later, in 1974, prominent nutritionist Dr Frederick J. Stare stated in a health guide that the average adult should aim for a daily fluid intake of 'somewhere around six to eight glasses per twenty-four hours'.[1] Importantly, he clarified that this fluid intake can come from a variety of sources, not just plain water. Beverages such as tea, coffee, milk, soft drinks, fruits, and vegetables all contribute to our daily hydration needs.

Over time, the nuanced recommendations regarding hydration were simplified into a rigid rule of 'eight glasses of water daily'. This oversimplification ignored the fact that hydration can come from multiple sources, including your morning chai or a bowl of watermelon. Yet, that original context remains both scientifically valid and physiologically relevant even today.

The body's hydration needs vary based on factors such as activity level, environment, diet, and individual physiology. Some people may need more, while others may need less. Our bodies have a remarkably sensitive thirst mechanism that works on autopilot and is the most reliable marker.

In fact, studies show that when your body's sodium levels rise, or when blood volume decreases, hormonal and neurological signals work in tandem to trigger thirst. I learned this intriguing information from a podcast featuring nephrologist Dr Joel Toeff, who discussed the mechanisms behind thirst and drinking water.[2] He explained, 'It takes about 10 minutes for the water that you drink to get into your bloodstream and your brain knows within a minute or so that you have consumed enough, and it is already like making the calculations based on what it is sensing in your mouth and your oesophagus.' This illustrates the complex mechanism our bodies use to detect and assuage thirst. Therefore, the notion that our body does not know if it is thirsty is simply incorrect.

That said, modern lifestyles can interfere with our body's natural systems, similar to how they affect our hunger and satiety signals. Many people spend long periods in air-conditioned environments, sitting at desks or in front of screens for hours, which distracts and disconnects them from their bodily cues. As a result, we might confuse thirst for hunger or suppress our thirst by drinking coffee, tea, or calorie-laden beverages instead. Over time, this can lead some of us to lose touch with our subtle thirst signals, making it especially important for older adults, as their thirst mechanism naturally becomes less sensitive with age.

While you do not need to force yourself to drink water by the hour, it is helpful to stay aware of your hydration needs. If your lips feel dry, your urine is darker in colour than pale yellow, or you have been active or exposed to the sun for a long time, make sure to hydrate yourself, even if you do not feel consciously 'thirsty'.

Temperature, Vessel, and Posture

Regardless of whether you prefer your water cold from the fridge, lukewarm, or at room temperature, rest assured that any of these options is perfectly fine. Your body will use the water just the same. While it is true that drinking cold water requires a small amount of energy to bring it up to body temperature, the calorie burn is too minuscule to make a meaningful difference in weight loss.

As for the type of container, whether it is a copper bottle, a steel tumbler, or a clay *matka* – it makes no difference to your hydration status. Copper bottles may release trace amounts of the mineral into the water, but these amounts are usually insignificant. The most important factor is that water should be stored in clean, hygienic containers.

Posture used while drinking – specifically whether sitting or standing – has become a surprising point of contention. Viral claims suggest that standing and drinking may lead to joint issues, kidney damage, or heart problems. However, none of these claims is supported by anatomical or physiological evidence. The position you choose to drink water in does not affect how your body processes it. Drink in a way that feels natural and comfortable for you.

Water and Weight Loss

Most weight-loss advice includes the recommendation to 'drink 2–4 litres of water a day'. While water does not directly burn fat or boost metabolism, it plays an important supportive role in weight loss. Staying well-hydrated can help regulate appetite and reduce unnecessary snacking, as we often confuse thirst with hunger. Choosing water instead of sugary drinks can also reduce overall calorie intake. That said, it is important to note that warm water does not 'melt fat', and cold water does not 'shock the system' into burning more calories. These ideas are oversimplified interpretations of much more complex physiological processes.

Putting It into Practice

Listen to your body. Pay attention to its cues. Drink water when thirsty, and do not worry about meeting an arbitrary number. Keep water within reach and sip throughout the day, especially when it is hot or when you are physically active. The temperature of the water, the container it is in, or whether you are sitting or standing matters much less than simply staying hydrated.

You've Got This

Your body instinctively knows when it needs water. The more we try to override its finely tuned systems with externally imposed rules, like reminder apps and marked water bottles, the more we risk disconnecting from our innate wisdom. Hydration does not require obsession; it simply calls for a little awareness and trust in how our bodies are designed.

3

Balancing Blood Sugar Throughout the Day

Welcome to the internet's latest pet obsession: glucose spikes. Influencers are now sporting continuous glucose monitors (CGMs) as fashion accessories, tracking every food-induced peak and trough, and creating daily content on Instagram featuring their food consumption, a CGM, and a graph of their glucose levels. But is this just a trend, or is it something we should pay attention to?

Let us explore.

What Is a Glucose Spike?

When we consume carbohydrates, digestive enzymes break them down into simple sugars, primarily glucose, which is then absorbed into the bloodstream. This postprandial (post-meal) increase in blood glucose signals the pancreas's beta cells to release insulin.

Insulin binds to receptors on insulin-sensitive cells, mainly found in muscle, fat, and the liver, facilitating the transport of glucose from the bloodstream into these cells. There, glucose can be used immediately for energy, stored as glycogen (mainly in the liver and muscles), or converted into fat if the body's energy needs are already met and glycogen stores are full.

This rise in blood glucose, followed by the release of insulin and the uptake of glucose, is a normal and essential physiological process. It is the body's efficient system for managing energy availability.

A 'glucose spike', in clinical and research contexts, refers to a rapid and substantial rise in blood glucose after eating. The size and speed of this rise are influenced by several factors:
- **Type and quantity of carbohydrate**: Simple sugars (like sucrose and high-fructose corn syrup) and refined starches (like

white flour) are absorbed quickly, leading to sharp increases in glucose levels. In contrast, complex carbs that are high in fibre break down more slowly, resulting in a slower rise in glucose levels.
- **Meal composition**: Meals that include fibre, protein, and healthy fats can significantly reduce post-meal glucose spikes. Fibre slows gastric emptying and glucose absorption, while protein and fat further moderate the body's response. A meal consisting solely of refined carbs will cause a greater glucose spike compared to a balanced meal.
- **Individual factors**: Various personal factors, including metabolic health, insulin sensitivity, genetics, gut microbiome, physical activity levels, sleep quality, and stress, can all influence how different individuals respond to the same meal in terms of blood glucose levels.

Why Glucose Spikes Matter

In the short term, people may experience mood swings, fatigue, increased hunger shortly after eating, energy crashes, or brain fog. These symptoms are often linked to a spike in blood sugar followed by a rapid decline. While occasional spikes are normal, frequent and intense spikes can put undue strain on your system and heighten the risk of chronic health issues.
- **Insulin overload and beta-cell burnout**: Repeated glucose spikes lead to frequent insulin release. Over time, this can overwork the pancreas, especially in genetically predisposed individuals, resulting in impaired insulin production.
- **Insulin resistance**: Chronically high insulin levels (hyperinsulinemia) can make cells less responsive to insulin, forcing the body to produce even more insulin, creating a vicious cycle that drives metabolic syndrome and type 2 diabetes.
- **Oxidative stress and inflammation**: A sharp increase in glucose can trigger oxidative stress and low-grade inflammation. Both conditions are associated with heart disease, cognitive decline, and even certain types of cancer.
- **Blood vessel damage**: High glucose levels, especially when paired with inflammation, can damage blood vessels and increase the risk of atherosclerosis, heart attacks, and strokes.

The Rise of the Glucose-Tracking Culture

The rise of CGMs among non-diabetics, along with glucose curve infographics and videos about taking vinegar shots before a meal, has helped highlight a key concept: blood sugar matters. However, this trend has also created hype and confusion. The goal should not be to flatten every glucose spike, as that is both unnatural and unnecessary. Instead, the focus should be on achieving metabolic flexibility: the ability to manage food intake, store energy, and switch between fuel sources with ease.

If you are active and metabolically healthy, indulging in an occasional sweet treat is perfectly fine. But if your diet leans heavily on UPFs, you are skipping meals, and you often feel tired, hungry, or irritable, it might be time to course-correct.

How to Balance Blood Sugar Without Obsessing over It

Forget fads and hacks. Here is what actually works:

- **The order of eating**: Start your meal with foods rich in fibre or protein, like a small salad, dal, or paneer, before moving on to rice or roti. This simple change in the order of eating food helps slow digestion and keeps blood sugar levels steadier after meals.
- **Prioritise protein at every meal**: Including protein in your meals promotes satiety, preserves muscle mass, and aids in blood sugar control.
- **Watch out for liquid sugar**: Be cautious with fruit juices, sweetened teas, and sugar-loaded coffees, as they can cause rapid spikes in blood sugar. Even a 'healthy' smoothie can have a greater significant impact than you might expect.
- **Move after meals**: Walking for just 10 minutes after a meal helps your muscles absorb glucose, significantly reducing blood sugar peaks.
- **Balance your carbs**: Choose whole grains, legumes, and vegetables instead of biscuits, white rice, or snacks made with refined flour. Adding fat or fibre can help reduce their impact.
- **Do not skip meals**: Long periods of fasting followed by carb-heavy meals can lead to dramatic spikes and crashes in blood sugar. Eating regular meals = steady energy.

Putting It into Practice

- **Balanced plate experiment**: At lunch, start with a small bowl of salad or stir-fried veggies. Next, add a protein (such as chicken, tofu, paneer, or an egg), followed by a grain (like rice, roti or millets which can be had with curries or dal). After two hours, check in with yourself to notice how your energy and focus feel.
- **Post-meal walk challenge**: After dinner, set a timer and take a 10-minute walk, either inside your home or around your building. Try this for three consecutive days and observe the difference.

You've Got This

Blood sugar management is not only important for those with diabetes; it is something everyone should be mindful of. You do not need a glucose monitor or to avoid foods like mangoes to manage your levels effectively. All you need is a little awareness and some simple adjustments in how you eat and move.

4

Protein Panic: How Much Do You Need?

As you scroll through your social media feed, the health-and-lifestyle gurus seem to be running a circus. One screams that you are a protein-starved skeleton doomed to frailty. Meanwhile, another claims that protein obsession is completely unnecessary and dangerous. Both flaunt their nutrition degrees, six-packs, and a million followers. And you cannot help but wonder, 'Whom do I believe, and how much protein do I actually need?'

In a world filled with protein water (yes, you read that right) and keto diets, protein has become more than just food; it is a lifestyle flex. Let us skip the spectacle and focus on the more important question: what does your body need to thrive?

The Science Behind Protein Needs

Protein is essential. It forms the building blocks of your muscles, organs, enzymes, hormones, and immune cells. But that does not mean 'more is always better'. Your body has specific requirements, and beyond a point, consuming excess protein will not build more muscle or increase your metabolism. Instead, that extra protein will simply be burned for energy or stored as fat.

How Much Do We Actually Need?

The Recommended Dietary Allowance (RDA) for protein is as follows: 0.8 g per kg of body weight per day for sedentary adults. That is about 46 g/day for an average woman and 56 g/day for an average man, both weighing 60 kg.

But here is the catch: that is the minimum required to prevent deficiency and not necessarily what is optimal for health, strength, or longevity. So, what do newer studies suggest?

- **For active individuals or older adults**: 1.2–1.6 g/kg is recommended to maintain muscle mass, support repair, and aid performance.
- **During weight loss or muscle gain**: Intake can safely increase to 2.0–2.2 g/kg/day depending on goals, although most people do not need that much in the long run.
- **For women during pregnancy or lactation**: Nutritional needs increase slightly over baseline due to the increased demand for tissue building and milk production.

It is important to note that protein needs vary based on age, activity level, metabolic conditions, and life stage, not gender stereotypes or diet trends.

Do Women Need Less Protein?

Women generally have less muscle mass on average, but protein needs are not determined by gender. Instead, they depend on factors such as body weight, activity level, and individual goals. The real issue is that many women are not getting enough protein. In cultures that glorify carb-heavy or low-calorie diets for women, protein often takes a back seat. Additionally, social pressure to eat small portions contributes to the problem, and it is no surprise that women end up under-fuelled.

Protein Quality and Timing

- **Complete versus incomplete proteins**: Animal sources (meat, eggs, dairy) offer all essential amino acids. In contrast, plant proteins (beans, grains) may lack some of these amino acids. However, smart combos like hummus with whole-grain bread or dal with rice can help fill in those gaps.
- **Spread it or stack it**: Traditional wisdom said your body could only use 20–25 g of protein per meal for muscle growth. A 2023 study published in *The Journal of Nutrition* challenged this notion, showing that consuming 100 g of protein in one meal can support muscle repair over a 12-hour period.[3] Eat what fits your lifestyle. Prioritise high-quality protein when it suits you best.
- **Leucine's role**: This amino acid triggers muscle repair post-workout. Aim for 2–3 g of leucine per meal, which is found in

whey protein, eggs, soy, and chicken. A scoop of whey protein or a tofu stir-fry post-gym does the trick.

Common Myths to Unlearn

- Myth: Consuming too much protein will damage your kidneys. Truth: For people with healthy kidneys, higher protein intake does not cause harm. This concern mainly applies to those with existing kidney disease.
- Myth: Plant protein is inferior to animal protein. Truth: While some individual plant sources may lack certain amino acids, having a variety of plant proteins in sufficient quantity can compensate for this.
- Myth: You need protein shakes daily. Truth: Protein supplements are convenient but not essential. Whole foods are perfectly capable of meeting your protein needs.
- Myth: Protein is only important for bodybuilders. Truth: Protein supports hormonal health, immune function, skin repair, and more. Everyone needs it, not just gym bros.

Putting It into Practice

- Front-load protein at breakfast. Ditch the sugar-loaded cereal and try eggs, paneer, Greek yoghurt, or a protein-packed smoothie.
- Plant-powered? Plan protein-rich meals by combining legumes, grains, soy, and nuts to cover all your essential amino acids.
- Post-workout? Prioritise protein with leucine. A scoop of whey (or plant-based protein, check labels), three eggs, or a tofu stir-fry will help maximise muscle repair.

You've Got This

Protein is just a nutrient – one piece of the puzzle that helps you feel strong and energised. The real question to consider is: 'Am I eating enough to fuel my life and achieve my goals?' That is the only protein flex worth caring about.

5

Whey Protein: Facts Over Fear

'Protein shakes are really bad! It takes three years to digest one scoop of protein shake.' These words, famously spoken by Ayushmann Khurrana on *The Ranveer Show*, left many science enthusiasts baffled.[4] Although it has been over five years since that statement, and he has since corrected himself, such myths about protein supplements continue to persist.

This is not entirely surprising. Even among well-educated Indians, including many medical doctors, there remains a widespread belief that whey protein and other supplements can be harmful to health, potentially damaging the liver and kidneys. Therefore, before dismissing protein shakes as dangerous or unhealthy, let us take a closer look at what whey protein actually is and address some of the most common misconceptions surrounding it.

Understanding Whey Protein

If you have ever made paneer or drained curd to make hung yoghurt, the liquid left behind is whey. It is a natural, high-quality protein source that your body absorbs quickly and uses efficiently. Whey contains essential amino acids, especially leucine, which activate the mTOR pathway to initiate muscle protein synthesis (MPS), essential for repair and growth. This rapid absorption makes whey ideal for post-workout recovery during the 'anabolic window' – the period after exercise when your muscles are especially receptive to nutrients for repair and growth.

Protein is a fundamental nutrient essential for the body's functioning. It consists of building blocks called amino acids and is best consumed as part of a balanced diet. Vegans and vegetarians must actively seek protein-rich options to meet their daily requirements. For elite athletes and individuals who work out to build muscle or burn high amounts of calories, meeting protein needs through diet alone can be challenging. This is where protein supplements, such as whey, can be beneficial.

Why Use Whey Protein?

- Helps meet daily protein requirements easily
- Supports muscle repair and growth
- Helps preserve lean muscle during weight loss by increasing satiety hormones like CCK and GLP-1
- Slows down signs of ageing
- Boosts skin, hair, and immune health through immunoglobulins and glutathione

Whey protein is a supplement, not a meal replacement. It is an add-on to your diet, handy on busy days, post-workout, or whenever you need an extra protein boost. It is especially useful for the elderly (to fight sarcopenia) and those with metabolic syndrome (to improve insulin sensitivity).

Choosing a Whey Protein Supplement

With so many types of whey protein available at varying prices, it is normal to feel confused about which one to choose. Here is a quick breakdown:

- **Whey protein concentrate (WPC)**: This contains around 70–80 per cent protein by weight and retains some fats, carbohydrates, and lactose due to less processing. It is a more economical option but may not be suitable for those with lactose intolerance.
- **Whey protein isolate (WPI)**: This has a higher protein content (90 per cent or more) and is processed to remove fats, carbohydrates, and most of the lactose. This makes it a good option for those seeking a high protein intake with minimal extra calories. It costs more than WPC due to additional processing.
- **Whey protein hydrolysate (WPH)**: Here, the whey undergoes partial hydrolysis, breaking down proteins into smaller units for easier absorption. It is typically the most expensive option and is popular for post-workout recovery due to its rapid digestion (within one to two hours).

Choose the variety that aligns with your dietary goals, lactose tolerance, and budget. Look for third-party tested products to ensure purity and avoid heavy metal contamination.

How to Consume Whey Protein

For optimal results, whey protein should be mixed with water and consumed within one to two hours after a strength-training workout. It is important to consume at least 25 g of protein with at least 2 g of leucine post-workout. If not part of your meal, whey protein supplements can easily help you meet this requirement. On non-workout days, whey protein can still be taken to help achieve your daily protein intake (aim for at least 1 g of protein per kg of body weight). Drink plenty of water while consuming whey protein, as a high-protein diet increases water requirements. Older teens and adults involved in sports or gym workouts can include whey protein in their diets, but it should not replace whole-food protein sources. If unsure, consult a doctor or nutritionist to determine a safe intake based on age, physical activity, and health conditions.

Should You Fear Whey Protein?

India faces an 80 per cent protein deficiency, yet a significant portion of the population fears increasing protein intake, especially whey supplements. Meanwhile, an entire alternate industry thrives on selling homemade laddus and powders as 'natural' alternatives to whey protein. These options are often very high in calories and contribute to the myth that whey is harmful. The belief that high protein intake damages the liver and kidneys has been debunked by scientific research. A 2016 study in *The Journal of Nutrition and Metabolism* observed athletes consuming a high-protein diet (3.3 g per kg of body weight) for a year with no adverse effects on kidney and liver function, lipid profile, or fat percentages.[5] However, individuals with pre-existing kidney conditions should consult a specialist before making dietary changes.

A Scoop of Caution

Although whey protein is generally safe, there are a few points to consider. Some people may experience mild digestive issues like bloating or gas, usually due to lactose intolerance. Opting for whey isolate instead of concentrate can help; however, some may still have problems even with isolate. As whey is derived from milk, it can trigger allergies in sensitive individuals. High protein intake can also affect medication absorption. Additionally, some people observe hormonal changes.

Counterfeit supplements or those adulterated with heavy metals, anabolic steroids, or herbal blends (like ashwagandha or green tea extract) can cause serious harm, including liver failure. Renowned hepatologist Dr Abby Philips has extensively discussed the safety of whey protein, emphasising that it is the adulterants – not whey itself – that cause liver injury.

Buy whey protein directly from brand websites or authorised retailers to avoid fake or contaminated products. Many e-commerce platforms have poor quality control. Being a largely unregulated industry, any company or factory can list supplements for sale.

Check labels for added sugar, as it can contribute to insulin resistance, weight gain, and metabolic issues.

Plant-Based Protein Powders

For those who are vegan or lactose-intolerant, plant-based protein powders made from pea, rice, soy, or hemp are good alternatives. However, it is important to note that most plant proteins are not complete proteins (meaning they lack one or more essential amino acids). To address this, many brands offer blended protein powders that combine different sources. Additionally, plant proteins vary in digestibility, and the processing methods used can influence their effectiveness.

Putting It into Practice

- If you struggle to meet your daily protein intake, consider adding a whey protein supplement to your diet.
- Choose one that fits your dietary needs and buy from a trusted source.
- Read the ingredient list carefully to avoid unnecessary additives, like sugar or herbal blends.
- Stay hydrated when consuming protein supplements to support digestion and kidney function.

You've Got This

Whey protein, when used responsibly, is a convenient and effective way to meet protein requirements, especially for vegetarians. Scientific evidence shows that it is safe for most people, and concerns about potential kidney or liver damage are largely myths. As with all supplements, quality matters. Choosing a reliable brand and using it in moderation can help you gain the benefits without any risks.

6

Fibre: The Unsung Hero of Your Diet (and Gut)

If fibre had a public relations agent, they would certainly need to be fired. In a world obsessed with protein powders and carb wars, fibre quietly does the grunt work without seeking any attention. It does not have a spotlight or hashtags, but it plays a crucial role in supporting our health with life-saving, gut-healing, inflammation-fighting ingredients. And yet, most people treat it like a dietary afterthought, if they think about it at all.

This is not just about avoiding constipation (though let us not pretend that it is not a big deal). Fibre is the foundation of your gut health, metabolic function, immune response, and, yes, even mental clarity. Ignore it, and you are not just skipping vegetables; you are ghosting the one nutrient that truly supports your body.

How Much Fibre Do You Need?

Let us discuss numbers. Most nutrition guidelines recommend consuming about 25–30 g of fibre per day. However, the average urban Indian only gets around 10–12 g, which is less than half of the recommended amount. This deficiency is largely due to the fact that whole grains, vegetables, fruits, and legumes – our primary sources of fibre – have been systematically replaced by white bread, biscuits, polished rice, sugary snacks, and a diet obsessed with protein over fibre.

Not One Fibre, But Many

Fibre is not a single ingredient. It is a family of plant-based compounds that work like a team. Understanding the types can help you get smarter about what goes on your plate: Soluble fibre helps lower cholesterol and regulate blood sugar. Insoluble fibre acts like a broom for your gut, sweeping away waste efficiently. Resistant starch feeds the good bacteria in your gut.

It is this diversity, not just quantity, that nourishes your microbiome and promotes long-term health. Once inside your gut, fibre does not simply pass through. The beneficial bacteria in your colon ferment undigested fibre into short-chain fatty acids like butyrate. These acids help reduce inflammation, support your immune system, and may even protect against colon cancer. In short, fibre helps foster the internal ecosystem that keeps you healthy from the inside out.

What About Psyllium Husk?

Psyllium husk (also known as *isabgol*) is a popular fibre supplement in India, and for good reason. It is a rich source of soluble fibre; just one tablespoon contains approximately 4 g. Taking two to three tablespoons a day can meaningfully boost your fibre intake, especially if your regular meals fall short.

It works well when stirred into water, smoothies, or yoghurt. But there is one essential rule: do not forget the water. Psyllium swells up by absorbing liquid, but without enough water, it can cause bloating or worsen constipation. Always take it with at least one full glass of water, and ensure your overall hydration is good. Fibre and water are a team; they work best together.

While psyllium helps with constipation and even cholesterol regulation, it is only one kind of fibre. Relying on it alone is like trying to meet your vitamin needs with only vitamin C – helpful but incomplete.

For long-term gut health, variety is key. A healthy gut needs different kinds of fibre, along with antioxidants and phytochemicals found in vegetables of all colours, fruits with skin, pulses, millets, nuts, seeds, and unprocessed grains. No supplement can match that diversity.

The Fibre Culture

Traditional high-fibre cultures, like Indian, Mediterranean, or Okinawan diets, do not treat fibre as a supplement; it is simply part of their meals. They include staples like rotis made from jowar or bajra, veggies with every meal, lentils, beans, fruits, and nuts.

By returning to our traditional eating habits, you can significantly increase your fibre intake.

Benefits of Eating a High-Fibre Diet

Fibre-rich foods are naturally more filling, aiding weight loss. They slow down digestion, blunt blood sugar spikes, and keep hunger at bay. If you have ever felt unreasonably hungry just an hour after eating a bowl of instant noodles or white bread, it is probably because your meal contained very little fibre.

Let us not forget the role of fibre in preventing lifestyle diseases. Several large studies have shown that people who eat more fibre have lower rates of heart disease,[6] type 2 diabetes, obesity[7], and even certain cancers.[8] The importance of fibre is often overshadowed by the hype around keto, gluten, superfoods, and the latest fasting trends.

Putting It into Practice

Before you chase the next miracle food or supplement, ask yourself: am I getting enough fibre?

I am not asking you to measure fibre by grams or buy anything special. Start by filling your plate with real food like vegetables, legumes, whole grains, and fruits. Add a spoonful of seeds. Snack on nuts. Let fibre co-exist on your plate as a guardian of your long-term health.

Here is what 25–30 g of fibre might look like in a day:
- A cup of cooked lentils or dal (15 g)
- One apple or pear (4 g)
- A handful of almonds or sunflower seeds (3 g)
- A bowl of oats with chia seeds and berries (8 g)

You've Got This

The wellness industry profits from your confusion, and fibre is just too straightforward to be highly profitable. It lacks celebrity endorsements, exotic origin stories, and complicated macro counts. Just fruits, vegetables, dal, seeds, and whole grains. Your grandmother's plate was probably a fibre-rich masterpiece, and we did not even realise it.

If you want improved gut health, glowing skin, hormone balance, metabolic strength, and even better moods, start with fibre. While it may not be flashy, it truly works. Let us give this unsung hero the recognition it deserves.

7

The Deficiency Myth: What Vegetarians Really Lack (and Don't)

'Hey *ghaas-phoos,* where will you get your protein from?'

You have probably heard it before, whether being said in passing or in mockery. You've even heard that vegetarians have all kinds of deficiencies.

It is the nutritional version of a concerned aunt or a dismissive uncle, casting doubt on your plate the moment it excludes meat. In wellness circles, vegetarianism is either glorified as a moral high ground or dismissed as a deficient diet, with very little space left for science or common sense.

Let us get this straight: vegetarians are not doomed to be iron-deficient, protein-starved, or perpetually weak. However, there are a few nutritional blind spots worth understanding – not because the diet is 'flawed', but because most diets, meat-inclusive or not, can lead to deficiencies when planned poorly.

What You Might Be Missing on a Vegetarian Diet

Vegetarian diets, especially in countries like India, can often be high in carbohydrates, consisting mainly of roti, rice, and dal, while lacking foods that provide essential micronutrients. These nutrient deficiencies typically result not from the absence of meat but from a lack of diversity and nutrient-dense foods.

Let us examine the most common areas of concern:

Vitamin B12

This is the big one. Vitamin B12 is found almost exclusively in animal products. A deficiency can lead to fatigue, nerve damage, and even cognitive problems. Even well-meaning vegetarians who 'eat healthy' often miss this because B12 has no reliable plant source. Some fortified foods, like nutritional yeast or plant milks, can help, but the safest route is a supplement.

Solution: Every vegetarian should have their B12 levels checked annually and take supplements accordingly. A simple methylcobalamin capsule or injection can prevent long-term damage.

Iron

Plant-based iron (non-heme) is not absorbed as efficiently as iron from animal sources. When combined with diets high in phytic acid (found in grains and legumes) or tea and coffee, which block iron absorption, the risk increases – especially for menstruating women.

Solution: Combine iron-rich plant foods like lentils, tofu, and spinach with vitamin C (like lemon juice or bell peppers) to enhance absorption. Also, avoid drinking tea or coffee immediately after meals, as they hinder iron uptake. Regular blood tests help detect low ferritin levels early.

Omega-3 fatty acids (EPA and DHA)

These heart- and brain-loving fats are primarily found in fatty fish. While some ALA (the plant-based omega-3 from sources like flax and chia) can convert to EPA and DHA (the active forms that support brain, heart, and eye health), the conversion rate is quite low.

Solution: Consider taking an algae-based omega-3 supplement, especially if you are pregnant, breastfeeding, or experiencing brain fog or dry skin.

Zinc

Zinc plays a crucial role in supporting immunity and aiding wound healing. However, its absorption can be lower on a vegetarian diet due to phytates found in plant foods.

Solution: To enhance zinc absorption, consider soaking, sprouting, or fermenting your grains and legumes to reduce phytate levels. Additionally, nuts, seeds, and dairy products are good vegetarian sources of zinc.

Protein

While vegetarian diets can absolutely meet protein needs, many people underestimate their intake or rely on low-protein staples. This is especially a concern for older adults or anyone pursuing strength goals.

Solution: To address this, be mindful of including high-quality vegetarian proteins like dairy, soy, lentils, beans, tofu, tempeh, nuts, seeds, and protein-enriched foods. Ensure that every meal contains a quality protein source.

Vitamin D

This is not just a vegetarian issue per se, but a modern living concern. Most people, regardless of whether they are vegetarian or not, are deficient in vitamin D because we are often not exposed to enough sunlight. Additionally, vegetarian or vegan diets frequently lack fortified dairy products or eggs.

Solution: Get your vitamin D levels tested and take a supplement if needed. Vitamin D3 derived from lichen is a suitable plant-based option for strict vegetarians.

Is a Vegetarian Diet Not Healthier?

Plenty of evidence links vegetarian diets with a lower risk of heart disease, hypertension, type 2 diabetes, and even certain cancers. But that is when the diet is built thoughtfully, not when it is an endless cycle of white rice, potatoes, and ultra-processed snacks.

A vegetarian diet rich in whole foods such as vegetables, fruits, legumes, whole grains, nuts, seeds, and dairy can be nourishing. However, when it is based on convenience foods or rooted in religious tradition without nutritional updates, the flaws become apparent.

Modern vegetarian diets, especially in India, suffer not from a lack of meat but from a lack of attention. When 'pure veg' becomes a moral identity rather than a nutrient-aware choice, deficiencies occur.

A Note for Vegans

If you are avoiding both dairy and eggs, you will need to be more strategic. Calcium, vitamin B12, and iodine can become low in your diet. Fortified plant milks, sesame seeds, ragi, and tofu can help provide calcium. B12 must be supplemented, as there are no reliable plant sources. Additionally, without egg yolks or dairy, your iodine intake may also become low unless you use iodised salt or seaweed in moderation. A vegan D3 supplement and an algae-based omega-3 might be worth considering, especially if you are often indoors or live in an area with low sunlight.

Putting It into Practice

- **Test, do not guess**: Have your levels of B12, iron (ferritin), vitamin D, and homocysteine checked annually.
- **Prioritise protein**: Ensure every major meal includes a solid protein source – like paneer, dal, soy, or yoghurt.
- **Supplement smartly**: B12 and D3 are almost non-negotiable in modern vegetarian diets. Algae-based omega-3s and occasional zinc might be worth discussing with your doctor.
- **Think variety**: Rotate your grains, pulses, and vegetables to introduce more diversity to meals. Fermentation and sprouting can increase nutrient availability.

You've Got This

The idea that vegetarians are destined for deficiencies is as outdated as the belief that cutting out meat guarantees better health. As with most things in nutrition, the truth lies somewhere in between. Instead of defending your food choices, focus on building meals that align your diet with your health goals – intentionally and intelligently.

8

Intermittent Fasting: What the Science Actually Says

Shrikant, a senior advertising executive in his early 40s, thrives on one hearty meal a day. He is a big eater, and this way, he can enjoy his food without worrying about calorie counting, snacking, or giving in to the canteen's Maggi and cheese toast. He feels clear-headed, energetic, and has managed to maintain his weight without obsessing over every bite.

Aarti, in her early 40s, works in publishing and has been experimenting with a 16:8 intermittent fasting (IF) routine. But her days are often dominated by food thoughts. She wakes up hungry, struggles with low energy and irritability, and ends up bingeing on comfort foods once the clock hits 'eating time'. Her initial weight loss plateaued, and now the process feels more discouraging than empowering.

The fasting camp claims it works magic, while sceptics argue it is just fancy branding for skipping breakfast. Both viewpoints have some truth. Intermittent fasting is one of the most polarising trends in modern nutrition. So is it a smart, science-backed tool, or just another passing fad?

Not a New Trend

Fasting is not some Silicon Valley innovation; it is ancient, rooted in Hindu, Christian, Buddhist, and Islamic traditions. It was about restraint, discipline, and seasonal renewal, not weight loss. Even our hunter-gatherer ancestors fasted, albeit unintentionally, when food was scarce. What is different now is how we view it. Instead of spiritual growth or survival, we fast for autophagy and abs.

So, What Is IF, Really?

It is a way of eating in which you voluntarily abstain from food for certain hours in a day or on certain days in a week. It does not prescribe what to eat, but when to eat. Some people combine it with a 'what to eat' approach by following a keto or calorie-deficit diet.

Here are the most popular IF methods:
- **Time-restricted eating (TRE)**: Fasting daily for 12 to 18 hours. The popular 16:8 method falls into this category.
- **The 5:2 diet**: Eating normally five days a week and limiting intake to 500–600 kcal on two non-consecutive days.
- **One meal a day (OMAD)**: All your daily calories are eaten in one big meal per day.
- **Alternate-day fasting or 24-hour fasts**: Some people fast completely (except water) once or twice a week.

How to Start IF?

The simplest way to start is to delay breakfast by an hour or two and eat dinner earlier. You sleep for seven to eight hours, so extending your fasting window during sleep is quite manageable. However, your morning masala chai habit may be affected. If it helps, substitute it with black coffee, green tea, or mint–tulsi herbal tea, all of which do not break your fast.

And when it is time to eat, how you break your fast matters. A protein-rich, savoury first meal like eggs, paneer bhurji, tofu stir-fry, or a bowl of skyr with seeds helps prevent the insulin spike that a sugary breakfast (cereal, toast, fruit juice) can cause after going more than 12 hours without eating.

Potential Benefits of IF?

IF has earned its moment in the spotlight for a reason. Some of the documented benefits include the following:
- Modest weight loss (mainly from eating fewer calories)
- Improved insulin sensitivity
- Reduced inflammation
- Mental clarity during fasting hours
- Enhanced cellular clean-up (autophagy) during fasting conditions

But let us be real: most human studies are short-term, small-scale, and often do not outperform simple calorie reduction. The flashy benefits you see in long threads on X, like fasting reverses ageing or melts visceral fat, are often extrapolated from studies done on rats or overhyped from early human data.

Autophagy, the cellular clean-up process that fasting supposedly boosts, is real but not exclusive to fasting. It also activates with regular exercise and quality sleep. And fat loss is basic calorie math. If you eat in a calorie deficit, you will lose weight, whether you fast or not.

The Flip Side: What You May Be Missing

Skipping meals also means missing opportunities to nourish your body. This matters even more if you are not a naturally big eater. If your daily protein requirement is around 80–100 g (which is typical if you are weight training or trying to maintain muscle mass), spreading it out over just two meals can be challenging, especially on a vegetarian diet, which often has more volume than a meat-based diet.

Most women struggle to reach their protein goals even across three meals, and eating all their food in a shorter window makes it even more difficult. Without adequate protein, you are not just delaying your fat-loss goals but also risking muscle loss.

This becomes especially problematic if you are also engaging in strength training. Your muscles need fuel, recovery, and regular protein intake throughout the day. Fasting for too long, combined with eating too little, can hinder strength gains, increase fatigue, and potentially raise cortisol levels, the stress hormone, especially in already-stressed individuals.

And let us not overlook the psychological impact. Constantly watching the clock, obsessing over the 'eating window', and managing cravings can increase food preoccupation, especially for people with a history of dieting or disordered eating.

So, Should You Do IF?

If it fits your lifestyle, does not cause stress or bingeing, and allows you to meet your nutritional needs, go for it. It is one of many tools in your health toolkit, not a silver bullet.

But if you are experiencing any or all of the following symptoms, then IF may not be your best bet right now:
- Waking up hungry and exhausted
- Skipping breakfast only to overeat at dinner
- Struggling to get enough protein or calories
- Losing strength or lean muscle
- Feeling irritable, foggy, or suffering from headaches

Putting It into Practice

You do not need to follow OMAD or 16:8 to see results. Even a 12-hour eating window (e.g., from 8 a.m. to 8 p.m.) allows for a metabolic break and is more sustainable for most people, especially women. Instead of strict fasting schedules, you could simply aim to avoid mindless evening snacking and improve your meal quality.

You've Got This

What is important is that your eating pattern supports your energy, strength, and performance instead of draining them. You do not need to fast like Twitter co-founder Jack Dorsey, who is known for his extreme fasting regimens. What matters is eating in a way that supports your goals and fits sustainably into your life.

9

Minimalist Eating: Why Variety Is Not Always the Spice of Life

Anita stands in front of her fridge and kitchen cabinets every morning, overwhelmed. Dozens of ingredients, a clutter of half-used condiments, and a stream of saved Instagram recipes leave her paralysed. She is exhausted by the mental gymnastics of planning three healthy meals every single day. Like many of us, Anita is a victim of choice overload.

Minimalist eating is a strategy that cuts through this chaos. It simplifies healthy eating by reducing decision-making and mental load. It is not an approach of deprivation or restriction, but a gentle recalibration of our relationship with food.

Minimising choices is not a new concept. Steve Jobs famously wore a black turtleneck and jeans every day to avoid decision fatigue. Queen Elizabeth, by many accounts, enjoyed a predictable menu, freeing up mental bandwidth for more important matters. These examples demonstrate a powerful truth: simplicity is a tool for efficiency, whether you are running a company, a country, or simply trying to take better care of yourself.

What Is Minimalist Eating?

At its core, minimalist eating is about shifting from living to eat to eating to live. In a society where food is associated with entertainment, comfort, and cultural identity, we often forget its primary role, which is to fuel our bodies. While there is joy in food, it should not overshadow its role as nourishment.

Minimalist eating promotes mindful selection of nutrient-dense foods, where each meal boosts your overall well-being. This often involves simpler preparation methods and focusing on whole or minimally processed foods that provide essential vitamins, minerals, and macronutrients. In many Indian homes, the idea of eating the same meals repeatedly is met with horror, especially when surrounded by a rich tapestry of regional cuisines and global food trends. But in a world obsessed with novelty, embracing a few favourites, nourishing meals can be revolutionary. Repeating meals streamlines your day, reduces waste, and frees up mental space. Imagine having three to four go-to breakfasts, lunches, and dinners that you truly enjoy and that align with your health goals. This consistency brings ease and predictability, turning healthy eating into a default habit instead of a daily challenge.

The Virtues of Minimalist Eating

While variety is often celebrated, it can also cause dietary chaos. The more ingredients, recipes, and food trends we add to our lives, the more choices we face, increasing the risk of decision fatigue and derailment.

Minimalist eating supports strategic variety – small, intentional changes within a core meal structure. Instead of having a completely different dinner every night, consider rotating grilled tofu, paneer, or chicken with roasted or stir-fried vegetables, changing only the spices or vegetables. This creates enough variation to prevent boredom while keeping you anchored.

Another benefit is emotional detachment from food. Not in the sense of being indifferent, but in freeing yourself from the emotional tug-of-war, where food becomes a reward, a distraction, or a coping tool. When you start to see food primarily as fuel, it lessens the emotional charge, helping you make clear-headed choices that align with your health goals.

It is important to understand that minimalist eating does not mean eating less. It is about organising your meals. You can enjoy satisfying portions of nutrient-rich meals while following a simple structure that fits your lifestyle.

For those who track their intake with apps, minimalist eating is a game-changer. Logging every new dish over a week can be tedious and unsustainable. But with a limited, familiar repertoire, tracking becomes faster, more accurate, and easier to maintain long-term.

A Caveat

Minimalist eating will not instantly resolve digestive or energy issues if there are underlying factors like gut dysbiosis, hormonal imbalance, poor sleep, or nutrient deficiencies. Additionally, for some individuals, overly repetitive eating may risk micronutrient gaps if not planned well.

So, while minimalist eating may indirectly support better digestion and energy by simplifying meals, reducing stress, and stabilising intake, it is not a cure-all. It serves as a gentle nudge towards more mindful, body-aligned eating.

Putting It into Practice

Start by selecting a handful of healthy meals you genuinely enjoy. Build these meals around whole foods, high-quality protein (plant- or animal-based), vegetables, whole grains, and healthy fats. Build your weekly meal plan around these, leaving room for small seasonal or flavour-based variations.

You've Got This

Embrace the simplicity and freedom of not having to decide what to eat every day. With fewer decisions, less waste, and more nourishment, you will start to see food as an ally instead of a source of stress.

10

Sugar: Friend, Foe, or Frenemy?

Sujata, 41, starts her day with a cup of filter coffee sweetened with organic powdered jaggery because she believes it is healthier than sugar. Her mid-morning snack is a 'clean' protein bar sweetened with dates, and her evening treat is a slice of banana bread made with coconut sugar. She completely avoids white sugar and feels virtuous in doing so.

What Sujata does not realise is that while she has ditched sugar, it still appears in her food throughout the day. She is not alone. Many health-conscious people today are swapping one kind of sugar for another, assuming they are making a better choice. But are they?

Let us peel back the labels to understand how sugar, in all its forms, impacts the body and how to make peace with it in a way that supports your health, energy, and sanity.

Our Relationship with Sugar

We grew up linking sugar with joyful things – birthdays, prasad, celebrations, post-exam treats. But as adults trying to take control of our health, we were told that this same sugar is the root cause of all evil. Soon, we began associating it with guilt, failure, addiction, weight gain, and a loss of control.

In the age of social media, sugar has been heavily vilified, with some influencers assigning it labels like 'poison' and 'toxin'. You have likely heard sugar being blamed for diabetes, PCOS, belly fat, 'toxins' in the body, and even cancer. It is no surprise that many of us have developed a fear of sugar but still consume it with apprehension or guilt.

The Truth About Sugar and Health

Refined sugar is a simple carbohydrate with no nutritional benefits besides energy or calories. Consuming too many sugary foods and drinks, especially ultra-processed ones, is associated with weight gain, poor metabolic health, dental problems, and increased inflammation in the body.

So yes, eating too much sugar regularly is not good for your health. But sugar itself is not the problem; it is the overall dietary pattern. If your day is filled with sugar-loaded chai, biscuits, mithai, and sugary cereals, and you are not getting enough fibre, protein, or healthy fats, then sugar does become a major issue. But eating a piece of birthday cake or a gaajar halwa after a wholesome meal? That is not what damages your health.

The Many Faces of Sugar

White sugar, or sucrose, is just one form of sugar. In the wellness world, it has been decisively cast as the villain. Instead, alternatives like jaggery, coconut sugar, honey, maple syrup, agave nectar, and date syrup have become more popular, marketed as 'natural', 'minimally processed', or 'nutrient-rich'. Some are even celebrated as superfoods. I am, of course, talking only about those who have the means for such choices. The vast majority can only afford regular white sugar.

It is true that jaggery or honey may contain traces of minerals or antioxidants. Coconut sugar has a lower glycaemic index because of inulin, a fermentable fibre. But when used in typical amounts – such as a teaspoon in tea or a tablespoon in baking (per serving size) – the nutritional benefit is negligible. No one should be eating jaggery for the iron or honey for its micronutrients.

From a physiological perspective, your body does not distinguish much between these sugars. In other words, your metabolism does not care whether your sugar comes from a fancy tree or a factory line; it treats them all the same. Agave's low glycaemic index might seem comforting, but its high fructose content can strain the liver over time, especially when consumed in excess.

A 2023 review in *Nutrients*[9] concluded that when consumed in similar amounts, most 'natural' sugars do not provide meaningful metabolic advantages over refined sugar. So while the type of sugar may slightly affect blood glucose spikes or insulin response, the bigger issue is how much sugar you eat overall, regardless of its source.

How Much Sugar Is OK?

Like alcohol, completely cutting out sugar from your diet is a good idea. However, it is not realistic or sustainable for most people beyond thirty-day challenges. The WHO recommends limiting free sugar intake to less than 10 per cent of daily calories, ideally under 5 per cent for added health benefits.[10] For most adults, this means no more than 20 g (about five teaspoons) of added sugar each day. But in India, the average urban intake is often double or even triple that, mostly from foods not perceived as sweet.

Processed breakfast cereals, commercial granola, flavoured yoghurt, nut butters, energy bars, ready-to-eat snacks, bakery goods, and sauces all sneak in sugar under dozens of names, such as brown rice syrup, maltodextrin, and fruit juice concentrate, to name a few.

Is Sugar as Addictive as Drugs?

The idea that sugar is as addictive as drugs has been around for years, but science does not fully support it. While sugar activates the brain's reward system, especially when combined with fat and salt (such as in caramel popcorn or gulab jamun), it does not lead to dependence or physical withdrawal symptoms like nicotine or opioids do. Often, what seems like a sugar addiction is actually a response to chronic restriction – when you tell yourself you cannot have it, you end up craving it even more. And when you finally 'give in', you tend to overeat it, which then reinforces the feeling that you are powerless around sugar.

Putting It into Practice

- Read labels carefully, not just the front of the package. 'Made with jaggery' or 'no added sugar' does not always mean low sugar. Learn to examine the ingredient list and nutrition panel. If sugar (or its many cousins) appears in the first three ingredients, it is probably a high-sugar product.
- Identify and replace one hidden source of sugar in your daily routine. Review your day-to-day diet and replace one sugary item – say, flavoured yoghurt or chai with sugar – with a lower-sugar alternative. This small change, repeated daily, can really add up.

- Give yourself full permission to enjoy sweets mindfully. Choose a favourite sweet and eat it slowly, without guilt. Notice how much you enjoy it when you are present instead of distracted or ashamed.

You've Got This

You are not failing if you enjoy a piece of chocolate or add a teaspoon of sugar to your chai. Sugar is not poison, and you do not need to fear every bite. With knowledge comes freedom. Learn to recognise excess, avoid hidden ingredients, and embrace the sweet things in life on your own terms, in moderation.

11

Fruit Fearmongering: A Wellness Trend Gone Wrong

It is bizarre that a juicy seasonal mango can spark the same level of panic as sugar-coated cookies among health and fitness enthusiasts. Ever since blood sugar, sugar spikes, and insulin resistance have become dinner-table conversation topics, fruits – especially sweet ones like bananas, grapes, and mangoes – are being viewed with suspicion. A frequently asked question these days is: is fruit just sugar?

Let us open that box of fruit and examine it.

Fruit Contains Sugar, It Isn't Sugar

When someone says, 'fruit is sugar', they are oversimplifying a nuanced truth about nutrition. Yes, fruit contains sugars, mainly fructose, glucose, and sucrose. But it also has fibre, water, vitamins, minerals, and an amazing variety of phytonutrients and antioxidants that play vital roles in cellular repair, immunity, and disease prevention – a combination that only nature can package so well. Compare this to a spoonful of refined sugar or a sugary soft drink that is completely lacking in nutrients, fibre, or what we call 'empty calories'. Whole fruit is anything but empty.

But What About Fructose?

In the war against sugar, fruit has sometimes been unfairly dragged in as collateral damage.

Fructose, the sugar found in fruit, has received a negative reputation in recent years, mainly because of research on high-fructose corn syrup (HFCS), an industrial sweetener used in UPFs and sugary drinks. The fructose in HFCS is absorbed quickly and in large amounts, burdening the liver and contributing to fat accumulation and insulin resistance when consumed in excess.

However, the fructose in whole fruit acts very differently in the body. Thanks to nature's smart design, the fibre in fruit slows down the release of sugar into the bloodstream. Fibre also helps with feeling full and supports gut health, both of which are beneficial for metabolic health.

To put it in perspective: you would need to eat about four to five apples to get the same amount of fructose as in one can of soda.

What Does Science Say?

A study found that even when participants with type 2 diabetes ate two or more fruits daily, it did not worsen their blood sugar control.[11] In fact, diets rich in fruit are consistently associated with lower risks of obesity, heart disease, type 2 diabetes, and certain cancers.

Population studies across the world, from Mediterranean to East Asian cultures, reveal high fruit intake as a common denominator in healthy, long-lived communities. So, why are we suddenly so wary of something humans have been eating for millennia?

The Rise of the Culture of 'Food Fear'

Much of the anxiety about fruit stems from social media wellness trends that oversimplify complex food science into categories of 'good' or 'bad'. People are told to never eat fruit after 6 p.m., avoid bananas at night or entirely because they 'spike blood sugar', or to never mix fruit with milk, dahi, or nuts. These blanket statements overlook context, individual health needs, and the overall quality of a person's diet.

Eating fruit as part of a balanced meal with protein and healthy fats is unlikely to cause a problematic glucose spike in most people. Even on its own, a piece of fruit is a much better snack than processed biscuits or energy bars posing as 'healthy'.

If you are insulin-resistant or managing prediabetes, working with a health professional to customise fruit choices (focusing on low-glycaemic index options like berries, apples, pears, watermelon, or guava) is useful. However, for the general population, there is absolutely no reason to fear fruit.

In the era of hypervigilance around food and nutrition, only berries seem to have been spared in the fruit world, leaving those of us in the tropics wondering if we can enjoy any of our beautiful local fruits at all.

A Few Fruit Facts to Remember

- **Timing is not everything**: Your body does not suddenly forget how to digest fruit after sunset. You can enjoy fruit at any time of day.
- **Do not overthink food combinations**: There is no scientific basis for rules like 'do not eat fruit with dairy'. A bowl of fruit with yoghurt and nuts makes a great snack or breakfast.
- **Juices are different from whole fruit**: Juicing removes fibre, concentrates sugars, and makes it easier to overconsume. Whole fruit is always the better option.
- **Frozen or dried fruit? Still good**: Just make sure there is no added sugar in the packaging. Frozen berries or dried figs retain most of their nutritional benefits. Remember that dried fruit is concentrated in sugars and calories, so eat them in small amounts.
- **Portion control still applies**: You can overeat anything, including fruit. But the threshold is much higher compared to ultra-processed snacks.

Putting It into Practice

- Aim to eat at least two to three servings of whole fruit every day, selecting a variety of colours and types across the week.
- Combining fruit with a source of protein or healthy fats gives more satiety and keeps blood sugar stable (e.g., banana + peanut butter + Greek yoghurt), but you do not have to do this all the time.

You've Got This

Let us stop vilifying fruit for being sweet. Yes, fruit contains natural sugars, but it also comes packaged with a suite of nutrients that support health rather than harm it. In the context of a balanced, whole-foods diet, fruit is your friend, not your enemy.

12

The 'Gluten-Free' Lie

Once upon a time, before health became a trending hashtag and your food choices were judged more than your morals, people ate roti without guilt. But somewhere between Instagram reels and supermarket aisles, gluten was crowned as the lead villain. The 'Gluten-Free' label, a badge of moral superiority, snuck onto everything, from almond flour cookies to shampoo. And just like that, wheat, a grain that nourished generations, was cancelled.

Most people avoiding gluten today don't have celiac disease. What they have is confusion – carefully packaged and sold to them by wellness influencers who have never set foot in a lab, by celebrities who mistake a bloated stomach for a diagnosis, and by food brands that know how to monetise fear.

Gluten is not the enemy. The narrative around it is.

What Is Gluten?

If you have kneaded dough to make roti or bread and left it to rest for a while, you would notice that the dough becomes elastic and stretchy, making it easier to roll out into rotis or shape into smoother loaves of bread. That is the action of gluten at work. It is a naturally occurring protein that gives dough its elasticity and chewiness. It is found in common staples like bread, pasta, chapatis, and bakery items made with wheat or refined flour. Unless you have been diagnosed with a condition that requires strict avoidance, such as celiac disease, gluten is not inherently harmful.

Should Gluten Be Avoided?

The popularity of gluten-free diets has stemmed from several sources. Celebrity trends and wellness influencers that promoted them as health solutions are one of them. Many people see improvements after cutting out processed foods, misattributing the benefits to gluten elimination. For others, the simple belief that they are making a healthier choice creates a placebo effect that feels like real improvement.

Scientifically speaking, gluten should be avoided only if you fall under these three conditions:

- **Celiac disease:** An autoimmune condition where gluten triggers damage to the small intestine. A lifelong, strictly gluten-free diet is essential here.
- **Non-celiac gluten sensitivity (NCGS):** A less well-defined condition where people experience digestive symptoms after consuming gluten, despite testing negative for celiac disease or wheat allergy. Symptoms may include bloating, brain fog, fatigue, or joint pain.
- **Wheat allergy:** An immune reaction to wheat proteins (not just gluten), requiring wheat avoidance.

These conditions cannot be self-diagnosed by watching videos online. They need lab tests, which may include a skin-prick test, blood test, or other complex tests. NCGS is a diagnosis of exclusion – if the person tests negative for celiac disease and wheat allergy but still has symptoms.

What Happens When You Cut Out Gluten for No Reason?

- **Nutritional gaps**: Eliminating entire food groups can have repercussions. Many whole grains that contain gluten, like wheat and barley, are rich in fibre, B vitamins, and essential minerals. Removing them without suitable replacements can decrease overall nutrient intake.
- **Dependence on gluten-free packaged foods**: Many gluten-free products are made with refined starches (like rice flour or tapioca starch) and lack the fibre or protein content of their whole-grain counterparts. These can spike blood sugar and are often more processed.
- **Unnecessary restriction**: Eliminating entire food groups without medical need can cause disordered eating or food anxiety.

People who genuinely need to avoid gluten must prioritise other whole grains, such as quinoa, millets, pulses, legumes, vegetables, fruits, nuts, and seeds, with minimal reliance on UPFs.

The Real Issue

Much of the discomfort people associate with gluten actually comes from eating highly processed wheat products like refined white bread, pizza crusts, packaged snacks, and biscuits. These foods are low in fibre, and high in sugar, salt, and additives, which can cause digestive sluggishness – not because of gluten, but because they are ultra-processed. Interestingly, traditional breads made with slow fermentation (like sourdough) may be better tolerated, even by some people with mild sensitivities. The fermentation process breaks down some of the gluten and FODMAPs (fermentable carbs), making them easier to digest.

Putting It into Practice

- If you do not have celiac disease or gluten sensitivity, you do not need to avoid gluten.
- Focus on decreasing ultra-processed carbs and adding more whole grains.
- Do not fall for gluten scare tactics. A whole-wheat chapati is not your enemy.
- Use your own body's response as your best guide. If wheat- or gluten-containing foods make you feel unwell, consult a doctor or dietitian to investigate the cause thoroughly.

You've Got This

Food has become a battlefield, and being healthy often feels like following a set of rigid rules. Gluten just happens to be caught in the crossfire. Let us choose common sense over fear when it comes to what we eat.

13

Which Cooking Oil Is Best for Your Health?

Let me clear up the great oil confusion right at the start. The quantity of oil you use daily is much more important than worrying about the types of oil that sit in your pantry. That might sound controversial in a world obsessed with labels such as cold-pressed, wood-pressed, extra virgin, organic, and so on. But it is the hard truth.

That said, understanding different cooking oils and their properties will help you make informed choices for various cooking methods. So let us dive into the details while keeping our perspective clear – moderation always trumps oil type.

Cold-Pressed Versus Refined: What Is the Difference?

The distinction begins with how these oils are produced. Cold-pressed oil is made by mechanically pressing seeds, nuts, or other source materials without applying heat. This preserves the oil's natural flavours, nutrients, and antioxidants, but results in lower yields.

Refined oil, on the other hand, is extracted using chemical solvents like hexane. After extraction, it undergoes neutralisation, bleaching, and deodorisation (because those solvents smell terrible), followed by filtration to remove impurities. This process yields more oil but removes some natural nutrients and antioxidants, resulting in a neutral flavour and lighter colour.

Is one inherently better than the other? Not necessarily. Each has its place in your kitchen.

Cold-pressed oils offer the following:
- More natural nutrients and antioxidants

- Distinctive flavours that can enhance your food
- Less processing and fewer chemicals

Refined oils provide the following:
- Better stability and longer shelf life
- Higher smoke points for cooking
- Neutral flavours that will not overpower your food
- Affordability

Traditional wood-pressed oil (known as *marachekku ennai* in Tamil) is similar to cold-pressed oil. It is made by pressing oilseeds between heavy granite stones, a method that does not use heat or chemicals and preserves nutrients and flavour.

Understanding Smoke Points

The smoke point is the temperature at which oil begins to break down and smoke. When oil reaches this temperature, it not only causes an unpleasant burnt flavour but also produces potentially harmful compounds. Here is a quick reference of smoke points for common oils (in Celsius):

Cold-pressed oils

- Extra-virgin olive oil: 190–210°C
- Light/refined olive oil: 240°C
- Avocado oil: 270°C
- Coconut oil: 175–200°C
- Flaxseed oil: 112–135°C (not suitable for cooking)
- Mustard oil: 190–200°C

Refined oils

- Canola oil: 204–232°C
- Peanut oil: 232°C
- Soybean oil: 232–266°C
- Vegetable oil blends: 204–232°C
- Rice bran oil: 232°C
- Sunflower oil: 232–246°C
- Mustard oil: 250°C

Using an oil beyond its smoke point is not just a flavour concern. It causes the breakdown of beneficial compounds and produces harmful fumes or free radicals.

Matching Oils to Cooking Methods

Different cooking methods require different oils. Here is a simple guide:
- **No-heat uses (dressings, dips, finishing)**: Cold-pressed oils are the best here. Their flavours and nutrients remain intact, and you will taste the difference in your salad dressings and dips. Try extra-virgin olive oil, flaxseed oil, cold-pressed sesame oil, or even cold-pressed mustard oil for a unique flavour.
- **Low-to-medium heat cooking (sautéing, light stir-frying)**: Both cold-pressed and refined oils with moderate smoke points work well. Extra-virgin olive oil, avocado oil, and coconut oil are good options.
- **High-heat cooking (deep frying, intense stir-frying)**: This is where refined oils with high smoke points excel. Peanut, canola, sunflower, rice bran, and refined mustard oils are the safest options here.

The Deep-Frying Dilemma

When it comes to deep frying, the three most important factors are smoke point, flavour, and cost.

Using cold-pressed oils for deep frying is like wearing designer clothes to paint a house – expensive and impractical. When you heat oil to 190–200°C for deep frying, many of the benefits of cold-pressed oils are lost anyway.

For deep frying, choose neutral-flavoured refined oils with high smoke points, such as rice bran, soybean, or peanut oil. Unless, of course, you specifically want coconut oil-flavoured banana chips.

Cost becomes significant when you are using expensive oils because deep frying requires large amounts of oil that typically cannot be reused multiple times. Avocado oil might have an impressively high smoke point, but it is not practical.

Regardless of which oil you choose, deep-fried foods should be consumed sparingly. Food fried in cold-pressed avocado oil will still have as many calories as food fried in refined oil.

Regular consumption can contribute to weight gain and chronic inflammation, no matter how 'healthy' the oil seems.

The Right Way to Reuse Oil

Oil begins to degrade when heated. While regular cooking methods like making dal or sautéing vegetables only involve heating oil once, deep frying leaves a significant amount of leftover oil, raising concerns about reusing it.

Repeatedly reheating oil produces harmful trans fats, free radicals, and polymers, collectively known as total polar compounds (TPC). According to FSSAI guidelines, oils should not be used more than three times, and those with TPC levels of 25 per cent or more should be treated as hazardous waste.

If you do need to reuse oil:
- Fry in small batches in a small pan to have minimal leftover oil.
- Strain cooled oil through a fine mesh.
- Store in a sealed container in a cool, dark place.
- Use this oil for lower-temperature cooking, like sautéing vegetables or making dosas, and not for deep frying again.

When disposing of oil, avoid pouring it down the drain or on the ground. Small amounts can be absorbed with newspaper and discarded in regular trash. For larger amounts, contact local restaurants or specialised recyclers who convert used oil into biodiesel.

Quantity Matters

Here is where we return to our initial point: the amount of oil matters more than the type. Even the healthiest cold-pressed oil can contribute to weight gain and health issues when consumed in excess.

Villainising refined oils while advocating everyone to switch to cold-pressed varieties often stems from a place of privilege. These premium oils are expensive and not affordable for all.

A more practical approach is to do the following:
- Reduce the total amount of added oils in your daily diet.
- Get healthy fats in their natural form from foods like coconuts, seeds, nuts, and avocados.

- Use cold-pressed oils where their flavours stand out, such as in dressings and low-heat cooking.
- Reserve refined oils for occasional high-heat cooking.

Putting It into Practice

- Use refined oils with high smoke points for deep frying, but only deep fry occasionally.
- Use cold-pressed oils either raw or with mild heating to maintain their benefits.
- Minimise consumption of oils in your daily diet, no matter the type.
- Prioritise reducing oil quantity over obsessing about oil types.

You've Got This

There is no one best cooking oil for good health. It is about using all oils wisely and in moderation. Your overall dietary pattern matters far more than whether your oil was pressed between granite stones or processed in a modern refinery.

14

Is Organic Food Just a Fancy Label or a Smarter Choice?

In this day and age, 'organic' has outgrown its exclusive image. What was once a luxury for the health-obsessed elite is now strewn across supermarket shelves and on every quick-commerce app. The Indian organic food market is projected to reach $8.9 billion by 2032, indicating that this is not just a passing trend. Even the same food corporations once criticised for pesticide-laden products are now offering 'organic-certified' alternatives.

But amid the certifications, eco-friendly packaging, and rising prices, one question remains: is organic food truly better for your health, or are we simply buying peace of mind in more attractive packaging? In this chapter, we look at what the science says, what the labels do not, and whether organic food lives up to the hype and the markup.

What Exactly Is Organic Food?

Organic food refers to food cultivated without synthetic pesticides, fertilisers, or genetically modified organisms (GMOs). It is the type of farming that our ancestors would have practised. Organic farming methods focus on the soil, nature, and surrounding ecosystems. Unlike conventional farming, which heavily relies on chemical inputs to maximise yield, organic farming employs crop rotation, compost, companion planting, and natural pest control to nurture the land. This results in food that is not only more sustainable but also, for many, more nutritious.

The Health Benefits of Organic Food

When it comes to eating healthily, organic food is often at the top of the list. But what exactly are the benefits, and are they worth the hype?

- **Higher nutrient content**: Scientific opinion is divided on whether organic foods are more nutritious than conventionally grown foods. A few reviews have concluded there is no real difference, but a large 2014 study analysed 343 research papers and found that organic fruits, vegetables, and grains had significantly more antioxidants, natural compounds that help protect our bodies from disease. Specifically, organic produce contained 20–70 per cent more key antioxidants, like flavonoids and anthocyanins, which are linked to a lower risk of heart disease, certain cancers, and brain-related diseases.[12]
- **Fewer pesticides and chemicals**: Conventional farming uses a variety of pesticides to protect crops, some of which have been linked to health problems such as hormone disruption and even cancer. Even after rinsing, pesticide residues can remain on your food. Organic food is free from these chemicals, making it a safer choice. The 2014 study also found that conventional crops had four times more pesticide residues and higher levels of a toxic metal called cadmium.[13]
- **No GMOs**: Organic farming prohibits the use of GMOs, unlike conventional methods that often rely on them. While GMOs are limited in India by law, with only Bt cotton approved, many consumers still prefer organic to avoid potential health and environmental concerns.
- **Better for animal welfare**: Organic farming also supports better practices in animal husbandry. Organic livestock are raised without antibiotics or growth hormones, both of which have been linked to various health issues in humans. This means less exposure to potentially harmful substances and more humane treatment of animals.
- **Taste and quality**: Many people claim that organic food simply tastes better. While this is subjective, organic food often has a more robust, authentic flavour because of natural farming methods that let produce grow at its own pace. Additionally, because organic farming focuses on soil health, organic food tends to have a richer nutrient profile, which can contribute to better taste.

Environmental Impact

Beyond your plate, organic farming has broader environmental implications.

Here is how it compares to conventional farming:
- **Soil health**: Healthy soil is the foundation of good food. Organic farming is gentler on the soil. Practices like permaculture, crop rotation, and composting help restore nutrients, which can improve soil structure and reduce erosion. Conventional farming, on the other hand, can cause soil degradation and depletion of essential nutrients, eventually making the soil less fertile in the long run and requiring more fertilisers.
- **Biodiversity**: Organic farms usually support a more diverse range of plant and animal life. Using fewer chemicals helps create a more balanced ecosystem, with a greater variety of pollinators, insects, and wildlife. Conventional farming often results in monocultures, which can harm natural ecosystems and reduce biodiversity.
- **Lower carbon footprint**: Organic farming practices require less energy and fewer synthetic inputs, which can help reduce their carbon footprint. However, yields can be lower, and more land might be needed to produce the same amount of food as conventional farming. This trade-off is an important factor to consider when evaluating the environmental impact of both systems.

The Cost Factor: Is Organic Worth It?

While organic food offers advantages, it also comes with a higher price tag. Organic produce can cost anywhere from 20 per cent to 50 per cent more than conventionally grown alternatives. The price premium is largely due to lower yields in organic farming, more labour-intensive methods, and the absence of government subsidies that often support conventional farming.

For those on a budget, start by choosing organic versions of the foods you eat most often, like fruits, vegetables, dairy, and meat. As demand for organic products continues to rise, prices may eventually decrease.

The Verdict

The debate between organic and conventionally grown food is complex. While organic food offers tangible benefits, such as higher nutritional value, fewer harmful chemicals, and more eco-friendly farming methods, it is not always the most practical or affordable option for everyone. Opting for local and seasonal produce, even if not organic, can still offer excellent nutrition and lessen environmental impact.

Rather than aiming for 100 per cent organic, aim for a balanced approach that includes a mix of organic and conventionally grown foods, based on your priorities, budget, and accessibility.

Putting It into Practice

Buy local, fresh, and from small, trusted farmers whenever possible. Organic produce in India can still have cross-contamination but residues are usually lower than in conventional produce.

You've Got This

You do not have to eat 100 per cent organic to be healthy. A diet rich in diverse fruits, vegetables, whole grains, and minimally processed foods, whether organic or not, will benefit your health.

15

The Whole Truth About Ultra-Processed Foods

A quick stop at a roadside shop in a city or tourist spot often greets you with garlands of chips, namkeen, or biscuit packets in bright colours. Even hospital canteens are not immune to this enticing display of packets of chips, sliced cakes, and biscuits, making it easy to grab a pack or two during your trip or hospital visit.

The scourge of UPFs has completely engulfed us over the years. We hear the term UPF constantly and might not pause to consider its meaning and implications.

Is Processing the Real Enemy?

Processing, in its foundational form, is not the real enemy. Basic methods like chopping, cooking, canning, freezing, and drying help turn raw ingredients into their edible and digestible forms. Canned vegetables, yoghurt, and pasteurised and toned milk are examples of this essential transformation, often improving food safety, nutrient bioavailability, and shelf life without fundamentally changing the food's molecular structure.

UPFs, on the other hand, are designed for hyper-palatability and extended shelf life. These food products undergo extensive industrial processing and contain several additives, preservatives, flavourings, colours, sweeteners, emulsifiers, and other ingredients. Some of these chemical interventions are designed to stimulate reward pathways and circumvent satiety signals in the brain, often making them addictive to consumers and highly profitable to sell. They are typically ready-to-eat or heat-and-eat and often come in bright packaging. Examples of UPFs include instant noodles and soups, sugary cereals, soft drinks, biscuits, namkeen, bakery and confectionery items, pre-packaged ready-to-eat meals, and many convenience items found in the centre aisles of supermarkets. Ultra-processed foods are often criticised for their potential negative impact on health due to their association with a range of health issues, including obesity, hypertension, metabolic syndrome, and other chronic diseases.

The Cascade of Health Implications

The scientific consensus is clear: UPFs lead to physiological disruption and disease.
- **Obesity**: UPFs hijack hormonal satiety signals, causing overeating and weight gain. The quick absorption of refined carbohydrates and the absence of fibre disrupt blood sugar regulation, leading to insulin resistance and fat storage.
- **Hypertension**: Their excessive sodium load contributes to an increase in blood pressure, thereby increasing the risk of cardiovascular events.
- **Metabolic syndrome**: They disrupt the delicate balance of metabolic pathways, leading to insulin resistance, dyslipidaemia, and accumulation of belly fat. The chronic inflammation induced by UPFs further exacerbates these metabolic disturbances.
- **Chronic diseases**: They drive systemic inflammation, a primary driver of cardiovascular disease, type 2 diabetes, certain cancers, and even mental health disorders. Artificial additives and the lack of essential nutrients contribute to cellular dysfunction.
- **Gut dysbiosis**: They disrupt the delicate ecosystem of the gut microbiome, compromising immune function and mental well-being. Artificial additives and the absence of fibre disrupt the delicate balance of gut bacteria, leading to inflammation and impaired nutrient absorption.
- **Addiction**: They trigger the reward pathways in the brain, creating a cycle of craving and consumption. The carefully calibrated combination of sugar, fat, and salt creates a powerful neurological response, leading to addictive-like

eating behaviours, making it difficult to stop at just one serving.

The History of UPFs

The manufacture and sale of UPFs date back to the mid-20th century. The post-World War II era witnessed significant changes in food production, driven by technological advancements and increased demand for convenience. Industrial processes enabled the creation of highly processed, packaged, and shelf-stable foods, marking the advent of ultra-processed products. They offered quick, but empty or nearly empty, calories to a working population.

Fast forward to 2025, the convenience offered by UPFs is unmatched for a busy lifestyle. Coupled with 10-minute delivery on quick-commerce apps, it creates a dangerous mix of poor nutrition and addiction.

Making the Change

Now that you understand what UPFs are and how they negatively impact our health, let me share the silver lining. The metabolic damage caused by these foods can be reversed by cutting back on UPFs.

- **Master reading labels**: This enables you to understand all that is in the packaged food and not blindly trust the claims made on the front of the pack.
- **Embrace whole foods**: Focus on fruits, vegetables, legumes, and whole grains. These are essential for cellular health.
- **Reclaim home cooking**: Do not think of cooking as a chore but as a way to best fuel your body. Take control of your ingredients and your health.
- **Limit UPF exposure**: Do not normalise UPFs as treats. Minimise their presence in your life and environment.
- **Let water be your main source of hydration**: Ditch sugary drinks, including those with low-calorie or zero-calorie sugar substitutes.

Putting It into Practice

- Gradually reduce the intake of UPFs rather than attempting drastic changes to make it easier and more sustainable over time.

- Practise mindful eating. Reconnect with your body's hunger and satiety signals. Treat eating as a conscious act of engagement with your body rather than a mindless activity.

You've Got This

Giving up UPFs is challenging but not impossible. It all comes down to restoring your body's natural equilibrium. Small, consistent changes form the basis of lasting transformation.

16

Reading Nutrition Labels: The Truth Behind the Packaging

My son had been advised by his doctor to avoid dairy temporarily, so we stocked up on almond milk as an alternative. Being an avid cook and a nutrition-centric health coach, I instinctively checked both the front and back of the almond milk pack. There was the unmissable label 'Plant Protein' on the front, a phrase that gives the impression of a protein-rich beverage. But when I turned the carton around, the label told a different story: just 1 g of protein per 100 ml. In comparison, cow's milk contains about 3 g per 100 ml.

That was a small but powerful reminder that if you regularly buy packaged foods and do not read the nutrition labels, you are probably being misled.

Why Nutrition Labels Matter

In recent years, the Indian food market has exploded with packaged options – from instant mixes and 'healthy' snacks to fortified drinks and ready-to-eat meals. Along with it has come a surge in marketing claims: 'low fat', 'natural', 'high fibre', 'zero sugar'. These labels are designed to catch your eye, not necessarily to tell you the truth.

Indian nutrition labels, while improving, still pose challenges. Some information is missing, ambiguous, or presented in confusing units. Yet learning to decode them is essential to making informed choices about what you and your family eat.

Front-of-pack claims versus back-of-pack reality

Front-of-pack claims such as 'high protein', 'zero fat', or 'multigrain' are often marketing tools. They can be legally used with minimal qualifying standards. For example:

- A product labelled 'high protein' may still contain less protein than you would expect.
- Almond milk may contain less than 1 per cent actual almonds.
- 'Multigrain' might indicate that several grains are present, but only in small amounts, with refined flour still being the main ingredient.
- 'No added sugar' may still include natural sugars, maltodextrin, dates, or sugar alcohols that affect blood glucose.

Always flip the package and read the nutrition panel and ingredient list.

Understanding serving size

Labels can be misleading when it comes to serving sizes. They often show values per 100 g or per serving.
- A pack may say '80 calories per serving', but one serving is defined as half a cup, while you are probably eating the entire cup.
- Always check the total grams or millilitres in the pack and do the maths if needed.

Ingredient list is where the secrets lie

Ingredients are listed in descending order of quantity. The first three ingredients reveal a lot about what you are actually eating. The ingredient list also shows the kinds of fats, sugars, and additives/preservatives used.

Look out for the following:
- Whole wheat bread where the first ingredient listed is refined flour or maida.
- Hidden sugars such as glucose, sucrose, fructose, or corn syrup, and maltodextrin.
- The presence of hydrogenated fats.
- Additives and preservatives: INS numbers, MSG, artificial colours, emulsifiers.

Even 'healthy'-sounding snacks or breakfast cereals can be sugar bombs with minimal fibre.

Know your nutrients

Here is a simplified cheat sheet to help you read common nutritional categories:

- **Calories**: Watch the serving size. A low-calorie label may only apply to a small portion.
- **Protein**: Look for at least 5–7 g per serving if it is a protein-based food. Some labels deceive us by inflating the protein content to include ingredients not inside the pack, like a high-protein muesli brand that counts the protein from 200 ml of milk added to the bowl of cereal.
- **Fats**: Focus on reducing saturated fat and trans fats. Ideally, trans fats should be zero.
- **Carbohydrates**: Subtract fibre from total carbs to get net carbs. High fibre (3 g or more per serving) is preferable.
- **Sugar**: Under 5 g per 100 g is considered low sugar. Watch out for sweeteners or hidden sugars.
- **Fibre**: Aim for high fibre intake; it helps digestion and keeps you full longer.
- **Sodium**: Under 120 mg per 100 g is ideal. Processed Indian foods often exceed this.

Do not be fooled by buzzwords

Here is a translation of common packaging jargon in Indian markets:
- 'No added sugar' – might still contain other sweeteners like dates or fruit concentrates.
- 'Low fat' – often compensates for high sugar or starch.
- 'Baked, not fried' – may still be high in carbs or fats from those added to the dough or base itself.
- 'Ayurvedic' or 'natural' – not regulated terms; these do not always mean healthy.
- 'A2' ghee – ghee is 100 per cent fat, while A2 is a protein that does not exist in ghee.

What to look for instead

- Short, recognisable ingredient lists are generally healthier.
- Whole grains, legumes, and seeds listed high up are a good sign.
- For meals or snacks, aim to balance protein, fat, and fibre.
- Brands that disclose complete ingredient breakdowns and honest serving sizes earn your trust.

Putting It into Practice

Reading nutrition labels is a skill. It does become easier with practice. In a world of confusing health claims and shiny packaging, this small piece of printed material helps you cut through the noise and choose what can truly nourish your body.

Labels are often designed to deter close reading, and some are in very fine print. Use your phone's zoom feature if needed!

You've Got This

In India, where regulations are constantly changing while consumer education struggles to catch up, being label-literate puts you at a distinct advantage. Whether you are grocery shopping for your child, managing a health condition, or simply trying to eat smarter, always read the back of the pack. If you shop online, most quick-commerce apps include a photo of the label in the product images, making it easy to review the ingredient list and nutritional information.

When it comes to your health, what is behind the box matters more than what is on the front.

17

The Best Cooking Methods for Everyday Meals

These days, every cooking method seems to come with a health warning. Fry something? Cancer. Microwave it? Radiation. Sauté with oil? Inflammation. The fearmongering is going out of control.

Ages ago, when 'cooking' was rudimentary at best for hunter-gatherer humans, meat was roasted on open fires and root vegetables buried in hot embers. Though they may not have been cooking in the refined way we understand today, those methods laid the foundation for all modern culinary techniques.

Fast forward to today, and we have a vast array of choices in our kitchens – steaming, sautéing, shallow frying, deep frying, air frying, baking, microwaving, pressure cooking, and more. With so many methods available, it is natural to wonder: which is the best way to cook our food?

The best cooking method is not a one-size-fits-all answer. It depends on the ingredient, the nutrients you want to preserve, and how well your body can absorb those nutrients. This concept is called bioavailability – cooking should not only retain nutrients but also enhance their absorption.

Let us explore some popular cooking methods, their pros and cons, and the best situations to use them for optimal nutritional benefit.

Steaming

One of the gentlest cooking methods, steaming preserves water-soluble vitamins like vitamin C and B-complex vitamins, which are easily lost in high heat or water-based cooking. Steaming is perfect for delicate vegetables like spinach, broccoli, and carrots. Unlike boiling, it does not leach nutrients into the water. Steaming also does not add any calories from fat to the food. Microwaves work well for steaming. Put your vegetables in a microwave-safe glass bowl with a splash of water. Cover with a silicone lid and microwave for three or four minutes, depending on the vegetable's requirement. If you steam for too long, the vegetables can become limp and soggy.

Sautéing

Sautéing in a small amount of oil not only enhances flavour but also improves the absorption of fat-soluble vitamins (A, D, E, and K) and antioxidants like beta-carotene and lycopene. For example, tomatoes sautéed in olive oil to make pasta sauce make lycopene much more bioavailable. When using cold-pressed oils, keep the heat low to moderate. Sauté vegetables for a short time to retain their colour, texture, and heat-sensitive vitamins.

Shallow frying

Used widely in Indian cooking, shallow frying can be delicious but should be used mindfully. It requires more oil than sautéing and hence increases calorie density. It is acceptable to use this method occasionally for certain dishes, such as tikkis or cutlets, especially when prepared with healthy oils and paired with vegetables or whole grains.

Deep frying

You do not need me to tell you this, but deep frying is the least healthy cooking method. As much as we romanticise eating vadapao or pakoras in the rains, regular consumption of deep-fried food is not a healthy option. High temperatures break down the oil, produce harmful compounds, and significantly increase the food's calorie content. Save deep frying for rare indulgences and avoid reusing the oil.

Air frying

This popular modern gadget mimics the crispiness of frying with a fraction of the oil. While not entirely oil-free, air frying is a better alternative to deep frying. That said, UPFs made in the air fryer are not automatically healthy. Use it to crisp up veggies or make protein-rich snacks, not frozen ready-to-cook foods like fries or nuggets.

Baking

Baking is a versatile dry-heat cooking method that is excellent for casseroles, vegetables, and protein-rich dishes. It typically causes minimal nutrient loss and is suitable for those trying to avoid excess oil. Roasting root vegetables in the oven enhances their natural sweetness and flavour without drowning them in fat.

Microwaving

Contrary to popular belief, microwaving is an excellent way to preserve nutrients, especially water-soluble vitamins, because of the short cooking time. It is also energy-efficient. Use minimal water and avoid plastic containers. Steaming vegetables in the microwave is both quick and nutrient-smart. It also be used to 'fry' papads or fryums without adding any extra oil.

Pressure cooking

No Indian kitchen is complete without a pressure cooker, and it is a staple in Indian kitchens for good reason. It significantly reduces cooking time and helps preserve nutrients that might otherwise break down during longer cooking processes. Although some sensitive vitamins may be affected by the heat, overall retention remains good, especially for pulses, legumes, and whole grains. Additionally, it aids in breaking down antinutrients like phytates, enhancing their bioavailability.

What About Raw Food?

Not everything benefits from cooking. Salads and fruits are best eaten raw to preserve vitamin C and enzymes. However, some vegetables like spinach, tomatoes, and mushrooms become more nutritious after light cooking because the breakdown of cell walls and antinutrients releases more nutrients. It is good to have a small portion of raw food alongside a variety of cooked food items.

Putting It into Practice

- Mix and match your cooking methods depending on the ingredient. For example, steam your broccoli, sauté your onions, and pressure-cook your dals.
- Do not fear cooking oils. Use them in moderation and avoid reusing them after deep frying.
- Vary cooking methods to prevent monotony and expand the range of nutrients.

You've Got This

You do not have to master every technique or obsess over losing a few milligrams of vitamin C. The healthiest food is not the most virtuous; it is the most sustainable for your lifestyle. A pressure-cooked dal, a sautéed sabzi, or a roasted sweet potato made in your own kitchen will always beat a sealed packet from a supermarket claiming to be 'clean'.

18

The Iron-Strong Plate: A Food-First Strategy for Anaemia

Anaemia is a silent epidemic – widespread, draining, and still surprisingly overlooked. The National Family Health Survey (NFHS-5, 2019–2021) reveals the harsh reality: 57 per cent of women (15–49 years), 67 per cent of children (6–59 months), and 59 per cent of adolescent girls in India are anaemic. Even one in five men in the same age group is not spared.[14] After decades of half-hearted campaigns and token supplementation efforts, the numbers remain staggering. How is a problem this widespread still treated like background noise?

Anaemia is leaving millions, especially women, chronically fatigued and struggling to function, while society dismisses it as 'just tiredness'. Enough with the apathy. It is time to stop patching the problem and start taking it seriously.

What is Anaemia and Why Does It Matter?

Anaemia is a condition in which your body does not have enough healthy red blood cells or haemoglobin to carry oxygen properly. The result is fatigue, dizziness, weakness, and low energy. In India, the most common form is iron-deficiency anaemia, but deficiencies in vitamin B12, folate, or chronic inflammation can also be causes.

This chapter mainly covers nutritional iron-deficiency anaemia because our diet (or lack thereof) can have a significant impact.

Nutrients That Help Prevent or Reverse Anaemia

To produce healthy red blood cells and sustain oxygen-carrying capacity, your body needs:

Iron: Vital for making haemoglobin. It comes in two forms: haem iron (from animal sources), which is easily absorbed, and non-haem iron (from plant sources), which needs help with absorption.
- **Vitamin B12**: Essential for red blood cell production. Found mainly in animal-based foods.
- **Folate (Vitamin B9)**: Helps in forming red blood cells. Found in leafy greens, beans, and lentils.
- **Vitamin C**: Boosts absorption of non-haem iron when consumed with iron-rich foods.

The recommended dietary allowance (RDA) of iron varies based on age, gender, and stage of life:
- **Adult men and post-menopausal women**: 8 mg per day
- **Premenopausal women**: 18 mg per day
- **Pregnant women**: 27 mg per day
- **Lactating women**: 9–10 mg per day

Foods That Help Combat Anaemia

Iron-rich foods
- **Haem iron (animal sources)**: Chicken, turkey, fish, and eggs are rich in haem iron, which is easily absorbed by the body.
- **Non-haem iron (plant sources)**: Lentils, chickpeas, tofu, spinach, fortified cereals, sesame seeds, Niger seeds, pumpkin seeds, coriander leaves, mint, and curry leaves are good sources of non-haem iron.

Vitamin C-rich foods
- Include citrus fruits (oranges, lemons), amla, guava, bell peppers, tomatoes, and broccoli to enhance iron absorption.

Folate-rich foods
- Dark leafy greens (spinach, curry leaves, moringa leaves), peas, beans, lentils, and avocados are packed with folate, helping support the production of red blood cells.

Vitamin B12-rich foods
- Eggs, dairy products (milk, yoghurt, cheese), and fortified plant-based milks (like almond or soy) can help prevent vitamin B12-deficiency anaemia.

Smart strategies to improve iron absorption
- Pair iron-rich foods with vitamin C sources in the same meal.
- Avoid tea, coffee, and dairy during iron-rich meals, as they can block absorption.
- Cook in cast-iron cookware to increase iron content naturally.
- Avoid consuming calcium-rich foods (like dairy) or caffeinated beverages (tea, coffee) during meals, as they can interfere with iron absorption.

Tests to Diagnose Anaemia

If you suspect low energy might be due to anaemia, your doctor may suggest:
- **Complete blood count (CBC)** to check haemoglobin levels
- **Serum iron studies** to assess iron stores (ferritin, transferrin saturation)

When Food Alone Is Not Enough

For mild to moderate cases, dietary changes can help significantly. But in cases of severe anaemia, especially if haemoglobin levels are below 10 g/dL, iron or vitamin supplements may be necessary.

These may include iron tablets, capsules, or syrups; vitamin B12 and folic acid supplements; or injectable iron in cases where oral supplements do not work or cause side effects. Always consult a doctor before starting supplements, as excess iron can lead to toxicity and other health complications.

Putting It into Practice

- Get a basic blood test (CBC) done annually, especially if you feel tired or follow a vegetarian diet.
- Get smarter with food combinations. Combine rajma–chawal with a kachumber salad of tomatoes, lemon juice, and bell peppers to boost iron absorption.

- Cook dal or sambar in a cast-iron pot.
- Do not pair your iron-rich meals with tea or coffee. Wait at least an hour after having tea or coffee to eat your meal.
- If your haemoglobin is low, talk to your doctor about the proper type and dose of supplements.

You've Got This

It all starts with what is on our plate. Awareness matters, but lasting change lies in the everyday choices we make. By prioritising iron-rich, nutrient-dense foods, we can do more than manage anaemia. We can reclaim our energy and bring real vitality back into daily life.

19

Alcohol: What Are You Really Toasting?

Recently, I saw a post on Instagram by an influencer that hit hard. It was a video recipe for a 'healthy' cocktail – kombucha spiked with vodka and a wedge of lime, calling it the best of both worlds. It struck me as the perfect metaphor for our generation's conflicted relationship with alcohol. We want the gut health, the glow, and the longevity, but we also want to hold onto the habit we have romanticised for years. Maybe it is time to ask: what are we really toasting to?

For many, alcohol has become a default setting – the celebratory clink of glasses, the social lubricant, ending the week with a long exhale. But when you step back and consider the real impact of alcohol on the human body and mind, the picture becomes far less enjoyable and much more sobering.

The 360-Degree Impact of Alcohol

- **The brain**: Alcohol is a central nervous system depressant. In the short term, it might seem to take the edge off, but what it does is decrease serotonin and dopamine activity in the brain, leading to increased anxiety and low mood the next day. Over time, this can increase the risk of depression and other mental health issues. There is also growing evidence linking alcohol consumption with cognitive decline and dementia.
- **The liver**: Among all the harms alcohol causes, its impact on the liver is perhaps the most widely recognised. The liver serves as our chemical processing plant, and alcohol puts it under great stress. Regular drinking leads to fat build-up in the liver (even in 'moderate' drinkers), which can develop into inflammation, scarring, and eventually cirrhosis. Once the liver is damaged, it triggers a domino effect affecting everything from digestion to detoxification.

- **Hormones and sleep**: Alcohol interferes with the endocrine system, throwing hormones like insulin, cortisol, and oestrogen off balance. It reduces REM sleep, increases nighttime awakenings, and dehydrates you, all of which means waking up groggy even after a 'full' night's sleep. For women, especially in perimenopause and menopause, the hormonal effects can worsen symptoms like hot flashes, mood swings, and sleep disruption.
- **Weight and metabolism**: Alcohol is calorie-dense and nutrient-poor. At 7 calories/g, it is just short of fat's 9 calories/g, but without the satiety or nutrition. It also spikes insulin, promotes fat storage (especially belly fat), and depletes your body of B vitamins, magnesium, and zinc, which are critical for metabolism. It also lowers inhibitions and increases the chances of making poor food choices. 'I will just have a salad' easily turns into 'Let's split a pizza' after a few drinks.
- **Cancer risk**: Here is something that people tend to ignore. Alcohol is a Group 1 carcinogen, falling in the same category as tobacco and asbestos. Even light to moderate drinking has been linked to an increased risk of breast, liver, colon, and oral cancers.[15] There is no safe threshold. That is enough reason to consider giving up alcohol completely. No level of alcohol consumption is safe for our health.[16]

But Is Red Wine Good for the Heart

The idea that wine (especially red wine) is 'heart-healthy' has been a powerful narrative, based largely on outdated studies that attributed the benefits to antioxidants like resveratrol.[17]

Animal studies indicate that a minimum of 500 mg of resveratrol is needed to get any health benefits (resveratrol supplements usually aim for 1–2 g/day), and it takes 40 litres of wine to get 500 mg of resveratrol!

The same cardiovascular benefits can be achieved through exercise, sleep, and a diet rich in polyphenol-containing plant foods, without the carcinogenic baggage. Also, relying on alcohol for antioxidants is as pointless as relying on a doughnut for dietary fibre.

The Social Layer

Giving up alcohol can feel socially awkward initially. People may question your decision, tease you, or make you feel isolated. But it is also incredibly empowering to say: I do not need this to enjoy myself, connect, or relax. What is more interesting is that alcohol-free living is gaining traction across all age groups. Saying 'I do not drink alcohol' is a flex like no other. There are now sober-curious circles, alcohol-free events, and amazing zero-proof drinks that do not mess with your hormones or your gut.

Putting It into Practice

- Try a 30-day alcohol-free reset. Do not just eliminate alcohol but also observe how your body responds. Track changes in your skin, sleep, digestion, mood, mental clarity, and energy. Your body will provide all the feedback you need.
- Replace the ritual. If alcohol helped you mark the end of a workday or the start of a weekend, establish new habits: herbal teas, a post-dinner walk, a playlist, journalling, or a glass of kombucha.

You've Got This

Alcohol has been marketed as pleasure, status, and even self-care. But once you stop drinking, you realise it was none of those things. It was just a pacifier, not a solution. This is not about missing out; it is about reclaiming your health with a single, powerful step: giving up alcohol completely.

20

Why We Eat When We Are Not Hungry

Roshni, 16, was studying for her board exams when she noticed a strange new habit: every time she felt stuck or overwhelmed, she would drift into the kitchen and return with chips or biscuits. The crunch and salt gave her a moment of comfort when the studies felt too much. It was not until she started journalling her study patterns that she saw it clearly: the snacking always happened when she was stressed.

Now, she keeps lighter snacks nearby, drinks more water, and takes short walks or plays with her dog between sessions. 'I still eat under stress sometimes,' she admits, 'but at least I know what is going on now.'

We eat for many reasons, and hunger is simply one of them. Sometimes it is stress. Sometimes it is boredom. Sometimes it is reward, comfort, nostalgia, loneliness, or just plain old, 'I have had a hell of a day, and I deserve this chocolate cake.' This is emotional eating. And if you have ever turned to food for comfort or distraction, you are not weak. You are human. And you are not alone.

What Is Emotional Eating?

Emotional eating occurs when we eat in response to our feelings rather than physical hunger. It is often prompted by emotions like stress, sadness, anxiety, frustration, boredom, loneliness, or even joy and celebration. For example, munching on popcorn at the movies not because you are hungry, but because it is part of the experience; having midnight ice cream after a hard day; or binge-snacking during study deadlines or exam season.

Food can make us feel better, but only temporarily. That first bite triggers the release of feel-good chemicals like dopamine and serotonin. It soothes, distracts, numbs, or energises. However, the relief is short-lived. The original emotion does not disappear; it just quietens for a while, only to return along with another craving.

Why Does It Happen

Emotional eating is not a lack of willpower. Instead, it is often a deeply conditioned response to stress or emotional discomfort. The origins can be traced back decades, even to infancy. The best way to calm a crying child is with milk. As children, many of us were comforted with food ('Do not cry, here is a biscuit'), rewarded with treats ('Let us go to the dentist, I will get you an ice cream after the appointment'), or guilted into eating everything on our plate regardless of our hunger ('Do you know how many kids go hungry in the world?').

We were not just fed; we were emotionally conditioned. Food became a language of love, reward, obedience, and even guilt.

Add to this the high-stress, low-sleep, fast-paced adult life, and food becomes one of the easiest and most accessible forms of self-soothing. Even more so with quick-commerce delivering food to us in 10 minutes.

Emotional Hunger Versus Physical Hunger

A good first step is learning to tell emotional hunger from physical hunger. Here is how they differ:

Emotional Hunger	Physical Hunger
Comes on suddenly	Builds gradually
Craves specific comfort foods	Open to a variety of foods
Feels urgent and impulsive	Can wait a little
Not satisfied even when full	Stops when you're full
Followed by guilt or regret	Ends with satisfaction

If you are reaching for a snack and wondering why, take a breath and check in with yourself: what is really happening here? Is it my body asking, or my mind?

The Consequences of Emotional Eating

The problem is not eating emotionally once in a while. That is a part of life.

When it turns into a regular pattern, it can:
- Disrupt hunger and fullness signals
- Lead to mindless overeating
- Interfere with digestion and sleep
- Delay or sabotage weight loss and metabolic goals
- Become a primary coping mechanism, reducing resilience over time

And worse, it does not actually fix the emotion you were trying to escape in the first place.

Steps to Break the Pattern

- **Start with awareness**: Keep a food and mood journal for a few days. Not to count calories, but to observe why you are eating. Note how you feel before and after meals or snacks.
- **Build a vocabulary for your feelings**: Often, we eat because we do not have a name or outlet for what we are feeling. Practise asking yourself: what am I really feeling right now? (Lonely? Anxious? Under-appreciated? Overwhelmed?)
- **Delay, not deny**: If you feel the urge to eat emotionally, wait 5 to 10 minutes. During that time, do something else – take a short walk, sip water, journal, or call a friend. This creates space between the trigger and the action.
- **Stock for success**: If you do find yourself eating for comfort, choose supportive foods. Keep fresh fruit, roasted makhana, hummus with veggies, or a handful of nuts nearby instead of sugar-laden, ultra-processed comfort foods.
- **Add, do not subtract**: Instead of only focusing on stopping emotional eating, focus on adding positive coping mechanisms:
  - Deep breathing or meditation
  - Physical activity (even five minutes of stretching)
  - Expressive writing or voice notes
  - Non-food rewards like a nap, music, or aromatherapy
- **Do not moralise food**: You are not 'good' for eating salad and 'bad' for eating a brownie. Food is not a moral issue. Let go of shame and show yourself some compassion.
- **Seek support**: If emotional eating feels unmanageable or is connected to anxiety, depression, or past trauma, consider

talking to a therapist who can teach you coping mechanisms to overcome it.

Emotional Eating Versus Disordered Eating

It is important to distinguish between emotional eating and eating disorders like binge eating disorder or bulimia. The latter involves a persistent, often uncontrollable cycle that impacts mental and physical health and requires clinical support.

If you suspect that your relationship with food is affecting your body image, mental peace, or day-to-day functioning, seek professional help. Catching issues early is better than struggling in silence.

Putting It into Practice

Create a 'comfort kit' to handle emotional eating. Instead of turning to food, prepare a go-to comfort box with a few of your favourite things. For example, a scented candle, a journal for your thoughts, a playlist of calming music, a soft blanket or stress ball, photos of loved ones or pets. When the urge to eat hits and you're overwhelmed by emotions, reach for your kit instead.

You've Got This

You do not have to turn into a mindful monk who never turns to food to soothe their emotions. Food will always have an emotional side, and that is okay. It can bring connection, joy, comfort, and nostalgia. It just should not be your only emotional outlet.

Part III

Built to Move

1. How Much Exercise Do You Actually Need?
2. Is Sitting Really the New Smoking?
3. Beyond 10,000 Steps: Make Walking Work for You
4. Strength Training: Not Just for Athletes and Gym Bros
5. No Crunches Required: The Real Science Behind Busting Belly Fat
6. Mat Versus Machine: The Great Workout Debate

1

How Much Exercise Do You Actually Need?

Some people spend half their waking hours at the gym, as if it is their full-time job, while others swear by their 30-minute home workouts, a bit of yoga, or a few walks each week. You'll find people from both camps on social media – one side sharing intense workout routines that feel like military training, and the other mocking gym-goers, claiming they are 'falling off like flies'.

If you have shown a passing interest in strength training, the algorithm assumes that it is your entire personality. Before you know it, your feed is filled with workout reels, ripped bodies, and whey protein ads. It seems like everyone but you is spending hours each day lifting heavy weights.

Drowning under deadlines, home chores, and social obligations, it is fair to ask: how much exercise is enough? Do you really need to spend hours at the gym to reap the benefits of movement?

The short answer: no. The longer, more useful answer: a carefully planned and consistent movement schedule is sufficient and far less demanding than you imagine.

What Qualifies as Physical Activity?

According to the WHO guidelines on physical activity and sedentary behaviour:[1]

> Physical activity is defined as any bodily movement produced by skeletal muscles that requires energy expenditure and can be performed at a variety of intensities, as part of work, domestic chores, transportation or during leisure time, or when participating in exercise

or sports activities. At the low end of the intensity range, sedentary behaviour is defined as any waking behaviour while in a sitting, reclining or lying posture with low energy expenditure.

Moderate-intensity exercises include brisk walking, cycling, swimming, and dancing. Vigorous-intensity exercises include running, high-intensity interval training, fast cycling, and sports like squash or football.

The WHO guidelines provide evidence-based public health recommendations on physical activity and sedentary behaviour for different age groups and populations, serving as an excellent resource for understanding how much exercise we actually need.

The Gold Standard: What Experts Recommend

This exhaustive and inclusive report contains evidence-based recommendations, and here is a summary:

Children and adolescents (5–17 years)

- Moderate-to-vigorous aerobic physical activity: at least 60 minutes per day.
- Vigorous-intensity activities and muscle- or bone-strengthening exercises: at least three days per week.
- Limit recreational screen time and overall sedentary time.

Adults (18–64 years)

- Moderate-intensity aerobic activity for 150–300 minutes per week, or vigorous-intensity activity for 75–150 minutes per week, or an equivalent combination. Spending 30 minutes daily on exercise, 5 days a week, is a good benchmark.
- Engage in muscle-strengthening activities at moderate or higher intensity for all major muscle groups on at least two days per week. This includes bodyweight exercises, resistance bands, free weights, machines, or activities like yoga and Pilates – anything that challenges your muscles more than usual.
- Limit sedentary time and substitute with physical activity of any intensity.

Older adults (65+ years)

- Same aerobic and muscle-strengthening recommendations as adults (18–64 years).
- Additionally, exercise like standing on one leg, tai chi, or yoga two to three times per week to reduce fall risk and improve coordination.
- Limit sedentary time by replacing it with physical activity of any intensity.

Pregnant and postpartum women

- Moderate-intensity aerobic activity: 150+ minutes per week.
- Incorporate various aerobic and muscle-strengthening exercises.
- Prior level of activity can continue if there are no contraindications.
- Limit sedentary time.

Adults with chronic conditions

- Individuals with cancer, hypertension, type 2 diabetes, or HIV should follow the above recommendations with required adaptations.
- Multicomponent activities are recommended for older adults with these conditions.
- Limit sedentary time.

People living with disability

- People with disabilities should follow the same recommendations with necessary adaptations.
- Physical activity offers additional benefits when tailored to different types of disability.

Important to Remember

- The guidelines stress that any amount of physical activity is better than none.
- People should start with small amounts and gradually increase frequency, intensity, and duration over time.
- The guidelines also emphasise that the benefits of physical activity outweigh potential risks for all population groups.

- Research suggests that, due to genetic and metabolic differences, South Asians may need approximately 230 minutes of moderate-intensity physical activity per week, i.e., about 80 minutes more than the standard WHO recommendation of 150 minutes. This translates to adding 10–15 minutes extra to your daily exercise routine. In simple terms, Indians need to work harder to achieve similar cardio-metabolic benefits as other populations.[2]

What If This Is Too Much for Me?

Do not think of exercise as punishment but as a celebration of what your body can do. If the earlier-mentioned guidelines feel like too much, do what you can because some movement is always better than none.

Just 10 minutes of intentional movement a few times a day can add up. Research shows that breaking up long sitting periods with light activity, like walking, stretching, or even dancing, can improve health markers such as blood sugar and circulation.[3]

Choose your exercise for the day based on your schedule, energy levels, and what makes you happy. Consistency comes easier when it does not feel like a chore or a punishment.

Building the Habit of Exercise

Start small and connect it to something you already do, like walking for 10 minutes after your morning coffee or doing mobility stretches before bed. Habit stacking (adding a new habit onto an existing one) works wonders. Consistency does not mean doing the same thing every day; it means showing up in ways that fit your life, again and again.

Exercise in Snack Form

No time for a full workout? Try a 'movement snack'. Just as we do not hesitate to reach for snacks when we are slightly peckish, we should not rely solely on one big workout session. Movement snacks, or short bursts of activity, help keep your body active throughout the day. Walk during phone calls. Do a few squats while you make your tea. Take the stairs when you can. These may seem small, but they add up, just like your unread emails.

Rest Days and Off Days

Talking about exercise without mentioning rest is not right. Rest is not laziness; it is a part of training. Muscles rebuild and get stronger during recovery. One or two weekly rest days help prevent burnout, soreness, and injury. Rest does not have to mean lying on the couch (though that is okay, too). A restorative walk, gentle yoga, or stretching counts as active recovery.

There will be weeks when things do not go as planned. Travel, illness, deadlines, and kids' school projects are a part of life. Missing a few workouts will not undo your progress. Just get back to your rhythm as soon as you can, and try not to miss two to three consecutive days, because that can become your new normal. Our body has impressive muscle memory and bounces back as soon as you return to your routine.

You've Got This

You do not need to spend hours in the gym or run marathons. All you need is a few hours a week, spread over the days, doing activities you enjoy, with a bit of motivation to keep improving.

A minimum of 150 minutes per week (around 21 minutes a day) is the recommendation. Feeling stronger, sharper, more mobile, and more in control is the payoff. Once you experience it, you will not want to stop.

2

Is Sitting Really the New Smoking?

'Sitting is the new smoking.' When Dr James Levine, MD, PhD, first coined this phrase, it may have seemed like an exaggeration. But research continues to confirm that extended sitting is connected to serious health dangers, making it one of the biggest silent killers of modern times.

'Sitting is more dangerous than smoking, kills more people than HIV and is more treacherous than parachuting. We are sitting ourselves to death,' says Levine, a professor of medicine at the US-based Mayo Clinic, in his book *Get Up!: Why Your Chair is Killing You and What You Can Do About It*.[4]

While the statement is provocative, some experts argue that sitting cannot be equated with smoking, since smoking has a direct, well-documented link to life-threatening diseases and causes passive harm to others. However, chronic inactivity has been clearly established as a cause of non-communicable diseases, making it a global public health concern.

How Prolonged Sitting Affects Health

The human body was never built to sit all day. Early humans spent most of their time walking, squatting, climbing, and running. In contrast, modern lifestyles demand long periods of sitting, whether at work, while commuting, or at home.

A sedentary lifestyle is a silent contributor to many chronic health problems. It increases the risk of type 2 diabetes, cardiovascular disease, high blood pressure, and metabolic syndrome. Staying inactive for long periods weakens key muscle groups, especially in the legs, glutes, and core. Blood flow suffers, increasing the likelihood of varicose veins and even deep vein thrombosis. Over time, a slow metabolism makes it harder for the body to control blood sugar and break down fats efficiently. Moreover, sedentary habits are closely associated with higher levels of anxiety and depression.

In India, this issue is especially severe. A 2014 study revealed that less than 10 per cent of Indians engage in recreational physical activity.[5] Since then, the rise of affordable internet, smartphones, remote work, quick-commerce apps, and endless streaming has only made it easier to remain sedentary and more difficult to stay active.

Why Exercise Alone Is Not Enough

While an hour of exercise at the gym or a daily walk is beneficial, it cannot fully offset the negative effects of sitting for the remaining 10+ hours of the day. This is why devices like smartwatches encourage users to move regularly throughout the day. Apple's Fitness app, for example, tracks three separate rings – Move, Exercise, and Stand – each playing a different role in lowering the risks associated with extended periods of sitting.

How Does Sitting Affect Your Metabolism

Just 30 minutes of sitting can slow your metabolism, lower calorie burn, and disrupt how your body manages blood sugar and fat. When large muscle groups, especially in the legs and core, remain inactive for long periods, they become less effective at moving glucose from the bloodstream. This gradual decline contributes to insulin resistance over time. Fat metabolism also decreases the activity of lipoprotein lipase, the enzyme responsible for breaking down fat for energy, which drops significantly during prolonged sitting, leading to increased fat buildup. Circulation also suffers as blood flow slows, raising the risk of swelling, blood clots, and decreased oxygen delivery to muscles.

Breaking the Sitting Cycle

Even small, frequent movements can undo the ill effects of prolonged sitting. Just five minutes of activity for every thirty minutes of sitting can help reduce metabolic slowdown. Here are some easy ways to add more movement to your day:

At work

- Take walking meetings instead of sitting in a conference room.

- Use the stairs whenever possible.
- Walk around while taking phone calls.
- Set a reminder to stand up every 30 to 45 minutes.

At home

- Break up TV time by standing, stretching, or doing squats during commercials.
- Do household chores like folding laundry or tidying up while standing.
- Walk around while talking on the phone instead of sitting.

On the go

- Choose public transport over cabs to incorporate more walking.
- If you drive, park farther away from your destination.
- Offer your seat to someone else on public transport and stand instead.
- Get off one stop early and walk the remaining distance.

Even seemingly small changes, such as standing during short tasks or using a higher desk to work in a semi-standing position, can have a noticeable impact.

On days when I take the Metro in Bengaluru instead of driving, I easily clock over 10,000 steps.

Putting It into Practice

- Avoid sitting for longer than 30 to 45 minutes at a stretch. Stand, stretch, or take a short walk.
- Look for opportunities to add movement to daily tasks instead of seeing them as inconveniences.
- Track your daily step count and aim for consistent movement throughout the day.

You've Got This

So, is sitting really the new smoking? Maybe not literally, but it has definitely become one of the most overlooked health hazards of modern life. Consciously break up long bouts of sitting by standing and stretching until it becomes a habit.

3

Beyond 10,000 Steps: Make Walking Work for You

My husband is an ultramarathoner who runs 250 km per race in some of the harshest conditions. I prefer the slower, steadier pace of walking. Whether I am reaching my step goal for the day or just clearing my head, walking is an essential part of my routine. I walk anywhere from thirty minutes to two hours a day while listening to podcasts, music, catching up with loved ones on the phone, or sometimes walking without my phone, experiencing the world around me.

Walking might seem too simple to be considered a powerful health tool, but research consistently shows it is one of the most effective and sustainable ways to improve overall well-being. Unlike structured exercise routines that need equipment, planning, or gym memberships (and money!), walking is accessible to almost everyone.

The best part? You do not need to carve out a lot of time for it. The goal of walking 10,000 steps a day, often cited as the gold standard, can be broken down into smaller segments. Walking your dog, taking the stairs instead of the elevator, strolling during work calls, or simply moving around the house for chores, all add up. Even on days I do not go out for a proper walk, I am often surprised to see I have logged nearly 6,000 steps just by staying active at home.

How Did 10,000 Become the Golden Number?

I was amazed when I learned this recently: the 10,000-steps-per-day goal did not come from medical science but from marketing! In the 1960s, a Japanese company launched a pedometer called the Manpo-Kei, which means '10,000-step metre'. The number was not based on scientific research but was chosen partly because the Japanese character for '10,000' looks like a walking person. It was memorable, catchy, and seemed like a reasonable fitness target.

Are 10,000 Steps a Day Necessary?

You do not need to hit exactly 10,000 steps to get health benefits. You do not have to chase that number. Even 7,000–8,000 steps daily can significantly lower the risk of cardiovascular disease and death. For older adults, even 4,000–5,000 steps daily show meaningful benefits.

Any increase in daily movement is better than none. Instead of obsessing over an arbitrary number, focus on moving more than you currently do, whether that is 5,000, 8,000, or 12,000 steps a day. Keep moving and do the best you can.

The Benefits of Walking

We all know that walking is good for us, but here is exactly how it benefits our health:

- **Reduces risk of heart disease**: Just 30 minutes of walking 5 times a week can lower the risk of coronary heart disease by 19 per cent.[6] The faster and more often you walk, the greater the benefits.
- **Boosts mental health**: Engaging in just 15 minutes of walking or running each day has been linked to a 26 per cent reduced risk of major depression.[7] Simply swapping 15 minutes of sitting for walking can boost your mood and ease stress.
- **Strengthens bones**: Postmenopausal women who walk at least a mile a day have higher overall bone density than those who walk shorter distances.[8] Walking also helps slow bone density loss in the legs, reducing the risk of osteoporosis.
- **Improves metabolic health**: Walking can counteract the effects of weight-promoting genes, curb sugar cravings, and reduce the risk of type 2 diabetes. A short walk after meals helps stabilise blood sugar levels.
- **Supports joint health**: Walking lubricates joints and strengthens the supporting muscles, reducing stiffness and pain, especially for those with arthritis.
- **Boosts immune function**: A study found that people who walk at least 20 minutes a day, 5 days a week, had 43 per cent fewer sick days than those who exercise less.[9]

How to Walk Smarter: Science-Backed Strategies

If you are already walking, great! But a few smart tweaks can help you maximise the benefits of the walks you take.

- **Walk first thing in the morning**: Morning walks before breakfast (or even before tea or coffee) can be particularly effective for burning fat. After an overnight fast, your insulin levels are low, making it easier for your body to access stored fat for energy. Even a 20-minute walk can be beneficial. Plus, it is a peaceful way to start the day, whether you use the time for reflection, listening to calming music, or simply enjoying the quiet.
- **Take a short walk after meals**: Taking a walk for 5–10 minutes immediately after eating can help control blood sugar and insulin levels. This is especially beneficial for those with prediabetes or diabetes. Walking right after a meal is more effective than waiting an hour, so plan accordingly.
- **2 per 20 rule**: If you work from home or have a sedentary job, you may sit for long hours without realising it. A meta-analysis[10] in *Sports Medicine* concluded that light walking for just two to five minutes every twenty to thirty minutes significantly lowers post-meal blood glucose and insulin levels compared to prolonged sitting. Simple strategies like walking around while on a call, grabbing a glass of water from another room, and doing a few stretches between tasks are useful. Even shaking legs or fidgeting counts as a small movement break! These tiny movements fall under NEAT, which makes up a significant part of daily calorie burn and metabolic health.
- **Walk outdoors for additional benefits**: While treadmill walking is effective, outdoor walks provide extra physiological advantages. Natural spaces are rich in negative ions, which help increase serotonin levels (the 'feel-good' neurotransmitter) and reduce cortisol (the stress hormone associated with belly fat).

Walking outside in the evening is an added bonus. Exposure to natural darkness signals the brain to produce melatonin, the sleep hormone. This results in better sleep quality, contrasting with the adverse effect of staring at a phone or laptop screen at night.

Walking at Any Age and Any Fitness Level

One of the greatest benefits of walking is that it can be adjusted to fit various fitness levels:
- **For beginners or older adults**: Start with gentle strolls, flat trails, and supportive shoes. If necessary, use a walking stick or rest frequently.
- **For those looking to intensify their walks**: Increase speed, incorporate inclines, or wear a weighted vest for extra resistance.
- **For those with mobility challenges**: Even small movements matter. Seated marching, pool walking, or simply moving your legs while sitting can help improve circulation.

Tech and Walking: Making It Fun and Gamified

Many people find walking more enjoyable when using step-tracking apps or smartwatches.
- **Step trackers**: Apps like Google Fit, Fitbit, or Apple Health can keep you accountable.
- **Gamification**: Challenges with friends, virtual races, or completing 'walking missions' (like exploring a virtual city) can add excitement.
- **Audio companions**: Podcasts, audiobooks, or walking meditations can make walks feel like productive time.

Putting It into Practice

If you are new to walking, start small: just 10 minutes daily. If you are already walking, try adding post-meal strolls (even inside the house), fasted walks in the morning, or nature walks for extra benefits. Every step counts. Often, the simplest habits lead to the biggest transformations.

You've Got This

Walking is often overlooked in favour of high-intensity workouts, but the science is clear. This simple activity is one of the most effective tools for lifelong health. It does not require special equipment, gym memberships, or extreme effort – just a comfortable pair of shoes and a willingness to move.

4

Strength Training: Not Just for Athletes and Gym Bros

For too long, strength training has been stuck in a stereotype of brawny men in sweaty vests, grunting through bench presses at gyms with walls full of mirrors. But here is a quiet shift in that perception. Strength training is for everyone who wants to build a body that works for them – one that is strong enough to carry your toddler, your groceries, or yourself into old age without falling apart.

You do not need to be an athlete. You do not need to 'bulk up'. You do not even need a gym. Strength training is one of the most effective tools to stay healthy, prevent disease, and move through life with energy and resilience. And it is for everyone, regardless of age, gender, or current fitness level.

Whether you are in your 30s trying to improve your posture, in your 50s aiming to stay mobile, or in your 70s working to prevent falls, it is about vitality more than vanity.

Let us explore how strength training fits into different stages of life and why it could be the most underrated health habit of all.

Strength Training Through Life (19–64 Years)

Benefits

- Increased muscle mass and strength, enhancing functional capacity and quality of life
- Improved basal metabolic rate, as muscle burns more calories than fat at rest, aiding in weight management and reducing chronic disease risk
- Improved bone density, reducing osteoporosis risk
- Enhanced cardiovascular health
- Stress reduction and improved mental well-being

Considerations

- Progressive overload (see Key Focus Areas later in the chapter) is crucial for muscle building
- Individualised programmes based on goals and fitness levels
- Proper technique and injury prevention are essential
- Balance strength training with cardio for overall fitness

Strength Training for Women

Women often worry that lifting weights will make them 'bulky'. The truth is, for women (or even men), building significant muscle mass requires a dedicated plan with high-calorie intake and structured training. For most women, strength training results in a toned, strong, and lean physique.

Strength training is particularly beneficial for women for the following reasons:

- Enhances bone mineral density, reducing osteoporosis risk
- Improves metabolic rate, aiding in weight management and body composition, especially during perimenopause and menopause
- Boosts mental well-being, reducing stress and enhancing body image

Strength Training for Older Adults (65+ Years)

As we age, strength training becomes non-negotiable. At this point, it is not just about looking fit; it is about maintaining independence, preventing falls, and staying mobile throughout life.

Benefits

- Combats age-related muscle loss (sarcopenia) and bone loss (osteoporosis)
- Improves balance and coordination, reducing fall risk
- Enhances functional independence and quality of life
- Reduces risk of chronic diseases (e.g., cardiovascular disease and type 2 diabetes) or slows their progression
- Improves cognitive function

Special considerations

- Prioritise functional exercises tailored to each person's limitations
- Start with low-intensity exercises and gradually increase the load
- Supervision by qualified professionals is highly recommended
- Focus on exercises that improve balance and stability

Children and Adolescents (12–18 Years)

Many parents ask: when is the right time for strength training? The early teen years are a great time to start, focusing on bodyweight exercises and mastering good form.

Benefits

- Enhanced bone mineral density, reducing future fracture risk
- Improved muscular strength and power, boosting athletic performance and functional capacity
- Enhanced motor skills and coordination
- Positive impact on psychological well-being and self-esteem, giving an early introduction to fitness and care for the body
- Injury prevention by strengthening supporting muscles and connective tissues

Considerations

- Begin with bodyweight exercises and perfect the form before adding weight
- Progress gradually, prioritising form overload
- Supervision by qualified professionals is essential
- Emphasise multi-joint exercises and a balanced approach
- Avoid excessive loading to protect growing joints

Key Focus Areas in Strength Training

- **Compound movements**: Exercises that work multiple muscle groups (e.g., squats, deadlifts, push-ups)
- **Lower body strength**: Engages large muscles like thighs and glutes for functional fitness
- **Full range of motion**: Promotes flexibility and prevents injury

- **Push-pull balance**: Prevents imbalances by training both sides of the body
- **Progressive overload**: Gradually increase stress on muscles to stimulate growth (via weight, reps, or sets)

Strength-Training Essentials: The Capsule Wardrobe of Exercises

You might feel overwhelmed by the wide range of complex exercises some trainers have their clients perform in the gym. In reality, you do not need all those complicated exercises. True strength training focuses on mastering a few key movements and progressively improving them. Here are the foundational exercises everyone should aim to master:

Lower body strength

Squats

- Excellent for lower body strength and stability
- Targets quads, glutes, and hamstrings
- Variations can accommodate different fitness levels (e.g., bodyweight squats, goblet squats, and barbell squats)

Deadlifts

- A compound exercise that engages numerous muscle groups
- Builds overall strength and power
- Requires proper guidance and perfect technique to prevent injury

Upper body pushing and pulling

Bent-over rows

- Strengthens the back and biceps
- Essential for postural support
- Can be modified with dumbbells or barbells

Bench press

- Targets the chest, shoulders, and triceps
- A staple for upper body pushing strength
- Variations include flat, incline, and decline presses

Overhead shoulder press

- Strengthens the shoulders and triceps
- Essential for overhead movements
- Can be performed with dumbbells or barbells (or lighter bamboo poles)

Lat pulldown

- Strengthens the back and biceps
- A good alternative to pull-ups for beginners
- Can be varied with grip width

Grip strength and core stability

Dead hangs

- Improves grip strength
- Helps with shoulder and spinal decompression
- Good for posture improvement
- Can gradually proceed to do pull-ups

Farmer's carry or farmer's walk

- Improves strength
- Anti-rotation exercise that helps with core stability
- Strengthens upper back and shoulders
- Functional fitness and real-life strength simulation
- Good for posture improvement

Bonus additions

- **Planks**: Builds core endurance and stability
- **Walking lunges**: Improves balance and single-leg strength
- **Calf raises**: Strengthens the lower legs and supports ankle stability

Choosing the Right Strength-Training Approach

The right coach or trainer

A good coach tailors programmes to your goals, prevents injuries, and helps with progressive overload.

Look for:
- Certified professionals (ACE, NASM, CSCS, or equivalent credentials)
- Trainers who approach your training with a proper plan, not random exercises thrown at you each day
- A coach who prioritises form and technique over simply lifting heavier

Apps, group classes, and community training

If you prefer self-guided workouts, apps can be helpful tools. Choose ones that feature video instructions to demonstrate proper form for each exercise, and those that can personalise the workout to match your fitness level and goals. Not everyone enjoys working out alone. Look for strength-training classes in your neighbourhood, which can be a good way to get started.

A few crucial points for strength training

- Always prioritise movement quality over quantity. Performing the movement correctly is more important than how much weight is lifted.
- Each exercise can be done with variations to accommodate different fitness levels and limitations. These are best taught by a qualified coach.
- Progressive overload is the principle of gradually increasing the challenge (weight, reps, sets) and is crucial for continued progress.
- Correct technique is of utmost importance to prevent injuries.
- Individual goals, limitations, and preferences should be kept in mind. Some may need modifications or alternative exercises.
- Always include a dynamic warm-up and static cool-down. When it comes to strength training, doing the same exercise with body weight or a lower-than-usual weight as the first set qualifies as a warm-up.
- Consult with a qualified healthcare professional or certified personal trainer before starting any new exercise programme.

When Is Strength Training Not Advisable

Strength training is not advisable for those facing one or more of the following issues:
- Acute injuries (fractures, sprains, post-surgery recovery)
- Severe cardiovascular conditions (unstable angina, uncontrolled high blood pressure)
- Severe osteoporosis (avoid high-impact loading; focus on controlled movements)
- Certain neurological conditions affecting balance and muscle control (work with a specialist)
- Uncontrolled diabetes (always consult a doctor before starting)

You've Got This

If you take one thing from this, let it be this: strength training is not optional; it is foundational.
- Start where you are. You do not need fancy equipment; your body weight is enough to begin.
- Progress slowly. Add weights, reps, or complexity over time. Find what works for you. Whether it is gym workouts, at-home training, resistance bands, or group classes, all of it counts.
- Make it a regular part of your routine. Strength training two to three times a week can significantly improve your long-term health. Your future self will thank you for this.

5

No Crunches Required: The Real Science Behind Busting Belly Fat

Do you remember when crunches were considered the holy grail for losing belly fat? I used to believe that too, until I realised the truth: you cannot spot-reduce fat. Crunches can tighten abdominal muscles, but they do not burn fat from the belly. Fat loss is a whole-body process, not something you achieve with a single move.

Why This Selective Bias Against Belly Fat?

For most people, the main reason is aesthetic. It is not just about preparing for the swimsuit round of Miss India or flexing their six-pack for Mister India. A flat midsection is often viewed as a sign of fitness. Clothes fit better. Even a ₹100 T-shirt can look like couture on someone with a flat midriff. But aesthetics, as the reason behind chasing the goal of a flat stomach, is barely scratching the surface.

Belly fat is not just one type of fat. There is subcutaneous fat, the layer of fat located just beneath the skin. Then there is visceral fat, the type that surrounds your internal organs. This second kind is more harmful, metabolically active, and disrupts your hormones. It increases inflammation and raises your risk of serious conditions like type 2 diabetes, heart disease, and some types of cancer.

A Bigger Problem for Indians and South Asians

Here is where things become even more relevant for us. South Asians, including Indians, have a unique body composition. We tend to have a higher percentage of body fat compared to Europeans, even at the same BMI. More importantly, this fat is disproportionately stored around the abdominal area. We all know that family member who looks slim but has a noticeable paunch or a friend with thin arms and legs but high cholesterol. This is the TOFI phenomenon: thin outside, fat inside.

Add to this epigenetics. Epigenetics studies how behaviours and the environment can cause changes that affect how your genes work. These changes do not alter your DNA sequence but influence how your body reads that sequence.

In India, generations of famine and undernutrition, especially during pregnancy and early childhood, followed by exposure to calorie-dense modern diets, have created a mismatch. Our bodies were designed to store fat as a survival mechanism, an evolutionary advantage that has now become a modern liability. So yes, your belly fat story is not just about what you ate last month; it is part of a longer history passed down through generations.

The good news is that epigenetic changes can be reversed with lifestyle adjustments, which brings us back to the original question.

Can Exercise Reduce Belly Fat?

While exercise can reduce belly fat, it doesn't do it in the way we once believed. The bad news: crunches won't give you a flat belly. The good news: you don't need them.

You should aim to move your way to better metabolic health. And as a bonus, a leaner waistline will tag along. Here is a seven-step, science-backed, and gentle programme to help you bust that belly fat.

Eat with a small calorie deficit

The only way to lose fat from anywhere, including the belly, is by consuming fewer calories than your body needs.

But here is where most people go wrong: they go too low. Starving slows your metabolism, tanks your mood, and sets you up for binge eating. And it is not sustainable.

Instead, aim for a modest deficit, around 300–400 calories less than your maintenance needs. Use an app like MyFitnessPal or a website like Calorie Calculator[11] to get a ballpark figure. Better yet, speak to a registered dietitian. You do not need to ban carbs or fats. Your body still needs all three macronutrients, carbs, protein, and fats, just in the right proportions.

Prioritise protein and fibre

Protein is your belly fat's most powerful opponent. Here is why:
- It keeps you full for longer
- It helps preserve lean muscle, keeping your metabolism humming
- It reduces cravings, which means less snacking on empty calories

Aim for 1.2–1.5 g of protein per kg of your ideal body weight. If your target weight is 60 kg, you need around 75–95 g of protein daily. Befriend foods like eggs, Greek yoghurt, skyr, tofu, low-fat paneer, lentils, and whey protein (if needed). Add chicken, fish, or other protein sources based on your dietary preferences.

And do not forget fibre. Fibre is your gut's best friend. It improves digestion, keeps you full, and has been linked to reduced belly fat over time. Include vegetables, fruits, whole grains, legumes, and seeds in your diet.

Movement, not just exercise

Strength training is your new best friend. It builds muscle, and muscle burns more calories at rest than fat. So the more muscle you build, the more fat your body burns, even while you are binge-watching your favourite show.

Start with bodyweight exercises like squats, push-ups, and lunges. Just two to three sessions a week can make a real difference.

And do not underestimate the power of NEAT. That is all the movement you do outside of exercise. Walking the dog, cleaning, climbing stairs, answering the doorbell, it all adds up.

Sleep deep

Many people believe that the road to fat loss is only diet and exercise. Sleep is often overlooked in the fat loss equation, even though it is foundational. If your sleep is as disturbed and limited as a new mom's, your belly fat will not go away. Poor sleep affects your hunger hormones, leading to cravings for more carbs and sugar. It also spikes cortisol, a stress hormone that is strongly linked to belly fat. Aim for seven to nine hours of good-quality sleep. Make it a priority over socialising, keeping up with the latest Netflix series everyone is talking about, or the IPL match.

Stress less

Managing stress, like getting enough quality sleep, is a passive approach compared with more drastic weight-loss measures. You can follow the best diet and exercise intensely, but if you do not manage your stress, your results will not be optimal. Chronic stress increases cortisol levels, which promotes visceral fat storage. Find what helps you unwind, whether meditation, journalling, gardening, singing, or playing with your dog. Even taking a few slow breaths between meetings can signal your body to relax. Your belly will thank you.

Watch your alcohol

I know it is tempting to unwind with a drink, especially after a long week, but alcohol is a triple whammy when it comes to belly fat:
- It adds empty calories.
- It impairs your sleep.
- It often lowers inhibitions and leads to overeating.

The less, the better. But if you do drink, track your intake and taper gradually.

Be patient, and play the long game

Fat, especially the stubborn kind around the belly, does not melt overnight. The body has its own schedule, and, unfortunately, it is not in sync with your wishful thinking.

Give yourself at least eight to twelve weeks of consistent effort before expecting visible changes. Do not let the mirror deceive you; progress often starts from within. All the steps outlined in this programme are making great contributions to your overall health.

You've Got This

You cannot just wish away belly fat, but you can outsmart it. For South Asians in particular, the stakes are high, but so is the power of lifestyle. When you eat smart, stay active, sleep well, and stress less, fat loss occurs, and your vitality comes back. No crunches needed!

6

Mat Versus Machine: The Great Workout Debate

Once upon a time, the gym was the shrine of fitness, where we all bowed our heads in reverence, praying to have the body of our dreams.

You either had access to a gym in your building or paid for a membership elsewhere, often hoping the hefty fee would guilt you into showing up.

Then came the pandemic, transforming living rooms into workout studios virtually overnight. Online coaches replaced in-person trainers, and simple equipment like yoga mats and resistance bands became the new essentials. Surprisingly, many discovered they preferred exercising at home.

Curious to understand how things stand in 2025 and the psychology behind people's preferences, I posed a question on X (formerly Twitter): 'Home workouts or gym workouts? What actually works for you and why?'

The responses came pouring in, revealing no clear winner. People held strong, with well-reasoned preferences for both options, highlighting an important truth: when it comes to fitness, no single approach works for everyone.

The Case for Home Workouts

Those who preferred home workouts listed several tangible benefits:
- **Efficiency**: No time spent commuting, waiting for equipment, or packing a gym bag. With fewer logistical hurdles, it's easier to stay consistent.
- **Flexibility**: You can work out whenever it suits you – before a meeting, after the kids are in bed, or even in your pyjamas. No fixed hours, no dress codes, no pressure.

- **Lower resistance to starting**: Not mental resistance, but that invisible force field between your bed and your gym shoes. At home, you just hit play on a video or unroll your mat.
- **Privacy and comfort**: Especially for beginners, working out at home removes the fear of being watched, judged, or overheard grunting through a plank. There is no 'performance pressure', which can be a huge relief.
- **Perfect for beginners**: With so many no-equipment bodyweight programmes available, home workouts are accessible to everyone, even those starting from scratch. Plus, you are spared the intimidation of watching gym bros deadlift your bodyweight five times over.
- **Some more reasons worth noting**: Home workouts are low investment. Your body weight is free. Resistance bands cost less than a month of a fancy gym membership. No pressure to dress up in branded athleisure either. Just roll out of bed, throw on mismatched clothes, and start moving before your brain realises what is happening. But it is not without cons.

Cons of home workouts

- **Progress can stall**: Bodyweight exercises only get you so far. Eventually, you will need resistance bands, dumbbells, or a gym setup to keep progressing.
- **Distractions**: Laundry, kids, phone calls, your dog thinking push-ups are an invitation to play; working out at home takes discipline and solid boundary setting.
- **Loneliness**: For some, working out solo can feel isolating and less energising.
- **Injuries**: Without a trainer or even a mirror, it is easy to slip up on form, and bad form leads to injury.

The Case for Gym Workouts

And then, the gym loyalists. Their reasons hit just as hard.
- **Structured environment**: The gym offers both tools and context. You are there to work out, and this psychological shift alone can boost your focus and performance.
- **Progression and variety**: Access to weights, machines, and group classes makes it easier to advance your fitness level and stay engaged.

- **External motivation**: Seeing others lift, sweat, and hustle can be motivating, especially if you thrive on social energy.
- **Trainers and support**: Having access to professionals who can correct your form or spot you safely is a big plus for both beginners and advanced lifters.

Besides these solid reasons, there is a lot of gym equipment that you simply cannot keep at home. And unless you are one of those rare people with a full gym at home, chances are you do not have a leg press machine or battle ropes lying around your bedroom. Also, sometimes, just watching someone deadlift twice your body weight is the kind of motivation you did not realise you needed.

Cons of gym workouts

- **Getting there is half the battle**: Commutes (hello Bengaluru traffic!), parking, crowds, waiting for machines, all of this can zap your motivation before you have even started.
- **Membership costs**: Not just money, but also the mental load of 'getting your money's worth'.
- **Lack of privacy**: For introverts and people who are self-conscious, exercising in a room full of strangers can be a barrier. 'Gymtimidation' is real, especially if you are new or feel out of place.
- **Overstimulation**: Loud music, bright lights, intense chatter, and people filming themselves for social media – some gyms can feel like sensory overload.

Enter: The Hybrid Era

The fitness landscape now includes options beyond the traditional home-vs-gym choice. Virtual training platforms offer expert guidance from the comfort of your home. Smart equipment tracks metrics and keeps you accountable. Apps deliver personalised programmes you can practise anywhere, from a hotel room to a park bench.

Hybrid approaches are becoming increasingly popular, with many combining gym and home workouts based on their schedule, energy levels, or life stage. This flexibility acknowledges that different environments meet different needs, and the 'best' workout space might shift over time.

Start with Your Goals

This is where it gets personal. Your ideal setup depends on what you want from your workouts right now. Ask yourself:
- What is your primary goal? (Muscle gain? Weight loss? Stress reduction? Just not turning into a couch potato?)
- What kind of environment keeps you motivated? (Solitude or social energy? Structure or flexibility?)
- What is realistically sustainable in your current life? (Time, kids, commute, budget?)
- Do you actually enjoy the activity, or are you dragging yourself through every session?

Looking to build serious muscle? The gym might give you better tools and progressive overload. Looking for flexibility and consistency? Home workouts may be the winner.

So What Is the Verdict?

There is no clear winner here. The better workout is the one you will actually do, regularly.

The goal is to move and build strength. Choose the format that feels manageable and can be done consistently in this season of your life. You do not have to stick with just one.

Do not let fitness culture make you feel guilty about thinking one path is better. You are not 'less serious' because you work out in your pyjamas. You are not crazy because you like deadlifting at 6 a.m. in a neon-lit gym. You are just someone who has found what works for them.

Exercise and movement are celebrations of your body, not punishments. Keep moving in ways that make you feel powerful. It is not about the location, but the habit. Consistency always wins.

Part IV

Your Home, Your Health

1. Airpocalypse Now: AQI 500+ and What to Do About It
2. Unfiltered Truths About Your Drinking Water
3. The Kitchen Is Where Change Happens
4. Do Not Fear the Frying Pan: A Sane Guide to Cookware
5. Plastic on Your Plate: The Kitchen Reality Check
6. The Gadget Gamble: Convenience Versus Wellness
7. The Hidden Toxins Lurking in Your Home and How to Send Them Packing

1

Airpocalypse Now: AQI 500+ and What to Do About It

Every October, as festival lights twinkle across India, another, less joyful season arrives in the National Capital Region (NCR) and spreads across North India: the season of toxic air. What was once discussed mainly by environmental scientists has become a topic at dinner tables, with terms like PM2.5, AQI, and air purifiers entering our everyday vocabulary. But behind the numbers and jargon lies a significant public health crisis.

Understanding the AQI Monster

The air quality index (AQI) measures multiple pollutants, among which the most harmful is particulate matter smaller than 2.5 microns (PM2.5). These microscopic particles cause the haze that often blankets the air and sky in the NCR region. They are small enough to slip past your body's natural defences, settle deep in your lungs, and even enter your bloodstream.

During the worst months, October through January, AQI levels in Delhi and nearby areas often exceed 400–500. For reference, the World Health Organization considers anything above 50 unsafe. Once you reach 500+, you are essentially smoking 25–30 cigarettes a day.

Why Does It Get So Bad?

A cocktail of factors creates this annual crisis. During winter, a layer of cold air rests close to the ground like a lid, preventing warmer, polluted air from rising and dispersing as it normally would.

Post-harvest stubble burning in neighbouring agricultural states sends large smoke plumes towards the NCR, making up as much as 40 per cent of the pollution during peak days. Vehicle emissions, construction dust, and industrial waste already keep the air poor before any seasonal factors even begin. Diwali fireworks, though increasingly regulated, can cause pollution levels to spike dramatically overnight, often pushing an already bad situation into hazardous territory. Open fires for warmth during the coldest weeks of winter, usually by the urban poor, add to the pollution load.

The Real Health Costs

Its impact on health extends beyond the immediate discomfort of burning eyes and scratchy throats. Here is what is really happening inside your body when the quality of the air you're breathing is poor:

- **Respiratory system**: The respiratory system is the most obvious target, with chronic bronchitis, asthma, and COPD (chronic obstructive pulmonary disease) all linked to long-term exposure to polluted air. Emergency room visits for breathing difficulties increase by 20–25 per cent during peak pollution months.
- **Cardiovascular health**: Less visible but just as serious is the impact of poor-quality air on your heart and blood vessels. PM2.5 exposure is linked to higher blood pressure, irregular heartbeats, and a greater risk of heart attacks and strokes.
- **Pregnancy and children**: Developing bodies are especially vulnerable. A study has shown links between air pollution and low birth weight, premature births, and developmental issues.[1] Children growing up in highly polluted areas show reduced lung capacity that may never fully recover.
- **Mental health**: Emerging research suggests connections between air pollution and higher rates of depression and anxiety,[2] as well as cognitive decline.[3] The ongoing stress of avoiding outdoor activities and worrying about your health also takes a psychological toll.
- **Long-term consequences**: A 2019 study suggested that residents of North India might be losing seven to ten years of life expectancy due to consistent exposure to hazardous air quality.[4]

Protective Measures: What Actually Works

While systemic change is desirable, personal protection is more achievable in the near term and has its own benefits.

- **Air purifiers**: These are no longer a luxury but a necessity. Select models with true HEPA filters and match them to your room size. Focus on bedrooms and living areas.
- **Effective masks**: Cloth and surgical masks are not sufficient. N95 or N99 masks, snugly fitted, offer real protection from PM2.5.
- **Create clean rooms**: Designate one sealed space in your home as a safe zone. Shut windows, use draft stoppers, and run your purifier there.
- **Indoor plants**: They help, but only slightly. Snake plants and peace lilies may reduce indoor pollutants, but they cannot remove PM2.5 during crisis-level pollution.
- **Air quality monitoring**: A home AQI monitor helps you track spikes and decide when to stay indoors or turn on the purifier. Some advanced air purifier models display PM2.5 or AQI levels.
- **Exercise timing**: If you need to go outside, early morning is usually the best time because AQI levels are lower. Check forecasts beforehand.

Your Indoor Air Sanctuary

While we focus on outdoor pollution, indoor air quality subtly impacts our daily well-being. We breathe in particles from cleaning supplies, furniture, and even walls. Here is how to turn your home into a true refuge:

- **Ventilation strategy**: Open windows for 15 to 30 minutes daily – when outdoor AQI permits – to reduce indoor toxins.
- **Smart cleaning choices**: Conventional cleaners with ammonia and synthetic fragrances emit harmful fumes. Switch to eco-friendly products or DIY solutions using vinegar and baking soda.
- **Avoid synthetic fragrances**: Air fresheners and scented candles release chemicals. Opt for essential oils or beeswax candles instead.

- **Humidity control**: Maintain humidity between 30–50 per cent to prevent mould growth and dust mites, while avoiding air that is overly dry.
- **Kitchen habits**: Always use exhaust fans while cooking. Gas stoves release nitrogen dioxide; avoid overheating non-stick pans.
- **Bedroom sanctuary**: Choose natural bedding materials and wash them regularly in hot water. Since we spend a third of our lives in bed, this matters significantly.

Beyond Individual Action

No mask or purifier can replace systemic change. Broader solutions include policy reforms with stricter emission standards, incentives for cleaner fuels, and sustainable farming practices. Community efforts, such as public air purification systems, carpool networks, and mass tree-planting drives, make a collective impact. Encouraging remote work on red-alert days can significantly reduce both emissions and exposure.

You've Got This

Living in high-pollution areas means balancing daily survival with long-term advocacy. The NCR's fight against the AQI monster offers a glimpse of what other cities may eventually face.

Start by creating one clean room in your home, like your bedroom or living area. Invest in an appropriately sized air purifier with HEPA filtration. Keep N95 masks handy for unavoidable outdoor exposure. Monitor AQI levels and adjust your activities accordingly.

Your home is your sanctuary, and you have the power to make it support your health. This is a fight worth fighting, and it starts with the air you breathe at home.

2

Unfiltered Truths About Your Drinking Water

Remember when 'drinking eight glasses of water daily' was considered revolutionary health advice? Now, we are navigating through tunnels of alkaline water, hydrogen-enriched water, structured water, and whatever new aquatic innovations Silicon Valley venture capitalists are funding next. Meanwhile, water filter companies are making billions by convincing us that our tap water might be dangerous, and bottled water corporations extract natural resources to sell us what should be a basic human right in plastic containers that will outlive our grandchildren.

But beneath the marketing hype and wellness influencer claims, there is a simple truth: water quality really matters, not in the way they are selling it, but in ways that truly affect your health and well-being. Let us explore this.

What Is in Your Water?

Municipal water supplies in most developed countries are regularly tested for harmful contaminants. Basic treatment removes pathogens and visible impurities, making it generally safe to drink. However, several concerning substances can still make their way into your glass.

Heavy metals such as lead and arsenic can contaminate water through ageing pipes or natural deposits. Even low-level chronic exposure has been linked to developmental issues, cardiovascular problems, and certain cancers.[5]

Chlorine and its byproducts, although essential for killing pathogens in water treatment, can form disinfection byproducts (DBPs) when they react with organic matter. Studies suggest potential links between long-term DBP exposure and bladder cancer.[6]

As the use of medicines grows, pharmaceutical residues are increasingly being found in water supplies. Although levels are typically very low, researchers continue to study the possible long-term effects of this chronic exposure.

Agricultural runoff containing nitrates, pesticides, and herbicides can seep into groundwater, especially in rural areas. Nitrate exposure is particularly dangerous for infants and pregnant women. Forever chemicals (polyfluoroalkyl substances or PFAS) from industrial processes are extremely persistent in the environment and in our bodies. Even minute amounts have been linked to hormone disruption, immune system suppression, and certain cancers.

Many places in India rely on groundwater (through borewells) or water delivered by tankers instead of municipal piped water systems, which can affect water safety. Borewell water often has high levels of fluoride, arsenic, nitrates, or other contaminants depending on the region. Tanker water comes from unregulated sources and may become contaminated during collection, transport, or storage. Neither of these typically receives the same level of treatment and monitoring as municipal systems.

Filtration: Separating Fact from Fiction

Not all water filters are made the same, and no single filter removes every contaminant. Understanding the technology allows you to make smarter choices.

Activated carbon filters (common in pitcher filters) improve taste and remove chlorine, volatile organic compounds, and some pesticides. However, they do not remove minerals, fluoride, or most heavy metals.

Reverse osmosis (RO) systems push water through a semipermeable membrane, removing almost everything, including beneficial minerals. They are effective but wasteful, usually discarding 7–15 litres for every litre of purified water.

Ion exchange filters are designed for specific contaminants, such as lead or arsenic, but do not address organic chemicals.

UV purification kills bacteria and viruses but does not remove chemicals or particulate matter.

The most effective approach often combines technologies, such as a carbon filter for chlorine and chemicals, followed by reverse osmosis for everything else, with a remineralisation stage to add beneficial minerals back.

Given these issues with water sources in India, selecting the right filtration method becomes essential to ensure safety and maintain water quality.

The Real Health Impact of Water Quality

Beyond the obvious risks of waterborne diseases, water quality affects health in more subtle ways.

- **Hydration efficiency**: Properly mineralised water (containing magnesium, calcium, and potassium) hydrates more effectively than pure H_2O, which is why athletes often choose electrolyte-enriched waters.
- **Mineral contribution**: Water can provide meaningful amounts of essential minerals like calcium and magnesium, particularly in 'hard water' regions. One study found that in areas where drinking water had higher magnesium content, residents experienced fewer cardiovascular deaths.[7]
- **Gut microbiome influence**: Chlorine in tap water may affect your gut bacteria composition. Some research suggests that chlorinated water might reduce microbial diversity in the gut, though more studies are needed.
- **Long-term exposure effects**: The body can manage occasional exposure to most contaminants, but decades of consuming even low levels of certain substances may increase the risk of chronic disease.

Finding Your Balance

For most healthy adults in areas with good municipal water, basic filtration like a carbon filter provides a good balance of protection and convenience. Those in higher-risk areas (with known contamination issues or ageing infrastructure) may need advanced systems like RO. In most urban homes in India, RO water filters have become the norm. Look for BIS (Bureau of Indian Standards) certified RO water purifiers.

The most crucial step is understanding what is actually in your water. Many utilities provide detailed water quality reports, and independent testing is relatively affordable if you have concerns.

Tailor your filtration system to your actual needs rather than falling for marketing-induced fears.

Putting It into Practice

- **Test and understand your source**: Check your water's TDS level (ideally 150–500 ppm) to inform filtration choices, especially important for borewell or tanker water, the consumption of which is common across India.
- **Maintain your filtration system**: Replace carbon filters every three months, clean storage tanks monthly, and inspect RO membranes annually to prevent bacterial growth and ensure effective filtration.

You've Got This

The solution for safe drinking water is not about special bottles, proprietary filters, or 'full moon vibrations', as some wellness influencers might try to make you believe.

The real solution is collective action to protect our water sources, update our crumbling infrastructure, and hold polluters accountable. While you figure out which filter fits your kitchen, big corporations are lobbying against clean water regulations and dumping industrial waste into watersheds that eventually reach your tap. Holding your municipal corporation accountable for water pollution is also essential for ensuring access to clean water for ourselves and future generations.

3

The Kitchen Is Where Change Happens

We are being sold the false idea that health comes from supplement bottles or trendy Ayurvedic wellness practices – that a healthy lifestyle means perfect smoothie bowls, organic everything, and a fridge straight out of an Instagram photoshoot. But the truth is far less glamorous and far more powerful.

True health starts with establishing certain systems. The science of behavioural change dictates that the environment you live in quietly influences every bite you take, every drink you pour, and every habit you repeat. Your kitchen is more than just a place to cook and do dishes; it is where your health is built or broken.

So let us stop obsessing over one-time meals and start building a solid foundation. One drawer, one shelf, and one decision at a time.

Make Healthy Choices Easier

Humans are visual creatures. Studies show that placing healthier foods at eye level increases the likelihood of choosing them.[8] The same reason is why retailers charge brands a premium to be at eye level, either in the store or in a prominent spot on their app or website. You can use this trick to help yourself eat healthier without much effort.

- Keep a fruit bowl on your kitchen counter.
- Store chopped vegetables or cooked lentils in transparent containers.
- Place healthy snacks, like roasted makhanas, spiced almonds, or seed mixes, at the front of the shelf, not hidden behind biscuit packets.
- Keep treats in opaque steel dabbas on a higher shelf that requires climbing on a chair to reach, or behind other healthier options on the shelf.

Beat the Decision Fatigue

One reason we often choose processed or packaged food is decision overload. When your kitchen is cluttered and chaotic, your brain tends to take shortcuts, usually opting for convenience instead of what is best for you. The simple solution is to reduce the chaos.
- Clear your counters. Keep only what you use daily – maybe a kettle, a cutting board, and knives.
- Organise your spices and staples. A labelled jar system not only looks good but also saves time and mental energy.
- Streamline your cookware. Keep only two to three high-quality, versatile pots and pans instead of a dozen mediocre ones.

Build a Cooking Rhythm

You do not have to meal-prep like a robot and eat the same meals all week. You can still prep by keeping a flexible structure that fits your real life.
- Cook in larger quantities when possible. A pot of dal or a batch of khichdi can be a lifesaver mid-week and is much healthier than ordering in.
- Chop onions, tomatoes, garlic, and ginger ahead of time and freeze in small portions. Use a food processor to handle the bulk chopping.
- Keep versatile ingredients on hand, such as cooked beans, cooked grains, yoghurt, shelled pomegranate, etc. These can be used in various meals.

The goal is to lower obstacles to real food and raise obstacles to foods you want to avoid.

Rethink Your Tools: Less Gear, More Usefulness

You do not need a gadget for every problem. In fact, having too many tools can cause confusion. The essentials include a sharp chefs knife, a good cutting board, a sturdy *kadai* or saucepan, a pressure cooker or Instant Pot, and a small blender for chutneys, smoothies, and masalas. Extras like an air fryer or food processor are helpful, but only if they fit your cooking style.

Make Hydration Easy

Dehydration often mimics fatigue or leads to unnecessary snacking. Make water the default beverage choice.
- Keep a water bottle or jug visible in each main room and a sipper at your work desk.
- Infuse water with lemon, mint, or cucumber if plain water feels boring.
- Avoid stocking sugary drinks. They cannot be a temptation if they are not in your house.

Light, Air, and Calm

Your kitchen does not have to be just a functional space. Lighting, smells, and sounds all affect how you feel when you are in it.
- Open the windows when cooking.
- Use task lighting or warm bulbs to make evening cooking pleasant.
- Play soft music or a podcast while you prep. It reduces the sense of 'chore' and brings in ease.
- Add some plants and hang some art in the kitchen to make it a visually pleasing space.

Make the Dining Space Sacred Again

If you eat on the couch, in bed, or while scrolling, you are not just missing out on joy; you are training your brain for distracted, disconnected eating.
- Set the table, even if it is just for yourself.
- Sit down to eat. Chew slowly. Breathe deeply. Digest properly. Take at least 20 minutes to eat a meal.
- Keep devices away from the dining area.

You've Got This

A healthy kitchen does not mean expensive, stylish, or Instagram-ready. It just needs to work for you. Arrange it to support your health goals. Come home, cook real food, and eat with mindfulness. That is health, right there on your plate.

4

Do Not Fear the Frying Pan: A Sane Guide to Cookware

In the quest for a healthier life, we often focus on ingredients – less sugar, more fibre, low sodium, organic products, and unprocessed foods. And then there is the worry about the pans we cook these ingredients in. It doesn't help that fear-mongering headlines (or influencers) are forever screaming that your non-stick pan is plotting to kill you, or that your cherished family heirloom aluminium pressure cooker is dangerous.

Somewhere between paranoia and indifference lies the sane middle ground. The truth is that cookware does matter, but not everything you hear about it is true. It is not about tossing out all your cookware or purchasing an expensive set of lab-tested pots. It is about understanding what each material does, when it might pose a risk, and how to work with what you already have.

The Real Science Behind Cookware Materials

Every material conducts heat differently and interacts with food in distinct ways. Some are completely safe when used properly, while others have real but manageable disadvantages. Let us explore them without panic.

Non-stick (Teflon/PTFE-coated)
- **Pros**: Uses less oil (beneficial for many people's health goals), easy to clean, great for foods like eggs or pancakes, less expensive than many other materials.
- **Cons**: Can degrade at very high temperatures (above 260°C/500°F), releasing fumes. Older coatings contained

PFOA (perfluorooctanoic acid, mostly banned now), which posed health risks.
- **Safe use**: Do not overheat an empty pan. Avoid metal utensils. Discard if the coating peels or gets scratched.

Cast iron

- **Pros**: Retains heat well, adds small amounts of iron to food (a bonus if you are iron-deficient), gets better with age when seasoned properly.
- **Cons**: Can rust, requires seasoning, and reacts with acidic foods if uncoated. Heavy pans may be difficult for older people to handle. Most quality cast-iron brands are expensive.
- **Safe use**: Season regularly. It is ideal for dry or high-heat cooking (such as searing or roasting).

Enamelled cast iron

- **Pros**: All the health benefits of cast iron without the rust or metallic taste. Safe for acidic foods.
- **Cons**: Heavy, expensive, and the enamel can chip.
- **Safe use**: Perfect for stews, soups, and sauces. Avoid metal spatulas. Fragile if dropped.

Stainless steel

- **Pros**: Durable, non-reactive, does not leach into food. Excellent for browning and deglazing.
- **Cons**: Can be sticky if not used properly (preheated and oiled well) and does not conduct heat evenly unless layered with aluminium or copper. Good-quality pans are expensive.
- **Safe use**: Versatile all-rounder. Use a heavy-bottomed pan for more even cooking.

Aluminium (including anodised)

- **Pros**: Excellent heat conductor, lightweight, affordable. Anodised versions are more stable and less reactive.
- **Cons**: Plain aluminium reacts with acidic foods, which can alter taste and leach trace metals.
- **Safe use**: Use anodised or coated cookware for everyday cooking. Avoid storing food in aluminium cookware.

Copper
- **Pros**: Heats very quickly and evenly, ideal for precision cooking.
- **Cons**: Uncoated copper can leach into food and be toxic. Most cookware is lined with stainless steel or tin (kalai). It is expensive and requires high maintenance.
- **Safe use**: If lined with stainless steel or tin, it is safe. Unlined copper should not be used for acidic foods.

Ceramic and ceramic-coated
- **Pros**: Non-reactive, smooth cooking surface, does not leach.
- **Cons**: Ceramic coatings wear out over time. True ceramic is safer but less common and more fragile.
- **Safe use**: Handle carefully. Replace when the surface wears off. Use low to medium heat.

Is Anything Actually Getting into Your Food?

Certain metals, such as iron, nickel, chromium, and aluminium, can leach into food in trace amounts, especially when cookware is damaged or used with acidic ingredients. However, in most cases, particularly with high-quality or well-maintained cookware, these amounts are extremely small and do not pose a significant health risk.

If you have specific conditions such as iron overload (haemochromatosis) or a nickel allergy, you may want to avoid cast iron or certain types of stainless steel. For most people, the main problem is not the pan but what is cooked in it. Cooking with reused oil, burning food, or loading up on processed sauces causes far more harm than any trace of metal leaching.

Choosing Cookware for Real Life

- For daily vegetables or stir-frying, use stainless steel, non-stick, or anodised aluminium cookware.
- For slow-cooked dals or sambars, use enamelled cast iron or stainless steel.
- For dosa or roti, use a well-seasoned iron griddle or cast-iron skillet.
- For tomato-rich dishes, use stainless steel or enamelled pans.

- For minimal-oil cooking, use good-quality non-stick cookware gently and avoid overheating.

You do not need ten different pans. A few carefully chosen ones, suited to your cooking style, go a long way.

Putting It into Practice

Start with a quick pan audit. Discard any non-stick cookware that is peeling or scratched. Give away the pans you never use (you know the ones). And when it is time to buy a new one, do your homework. Match the type of pan to your cooking style and invest in the best quality your budget allows.

You've Got This

Here is the thing no cookware company will tell you: your health relies far more on your habits than on your equipment.

The pan matters, but it is not a moral decision. Stainless steel is not sacred, and non-stick is not evil. What matters more is whether you are cooking at home in the first place, if you are steaming vegetables instead of ordering fries, if you are making dal instead of tearing open an instant soup packet.

Do not fear your pan. The healthiest kitchen is not the one with the fanciest cookware, but the one where food is prepared with care and real ingredients.

5

Plastic on Your Plate: The Kitchen Reality Check

Many of us grew up in households where the kitchen was a museum of mismatched plasticware. The fridge was full of surprises. Open an ice cream tub and, surprise, it has coriander inside. Reach for the cheese spread, and you've instead found a lone half-cut lemon. You get the idea.

Fast forward to today, and you hear things on the internet like: 'If you are what you eat, then I am plastic.' It sounds absurd until you realise it might not be far from the truth. Research suggests we may be ingesting up to 5 g of microplastics a week, the equivalent of a credit card, through food, water, and even the air we breathe.

As usual, this conversation has been taken over by guilt and Instagram aesthetics. You are told your kitchen should look like a zero-waste art installation with glass jars, bamboo lids, and terracotta everything. But here are some truths: not all plastic is toxic; not all non-plastic is safe. Switching materials just for appearances is emerging as a new kind of superstition.

What Science Really Says

Most plastic kitchenware is made from polymers like polyethylene or polypropylene. These base materials are not inherently toxic. The concern comes from what is added to them. For example, chemicals like BPA, phthalates, and other additives that can leach into food. These are endocrine disruptors, which means they can interfere with hormone function, potentially affecting fertility, metabolism, and long-term disease risk.

Microplastics are tiny particles less than 5 mm in size, shed from plastic packaging and utensils. These particles have been detected in human blood,[9] lungs, and arterial plaques. One 2024 study even linked their presence in arteries with a higher risk of heart attacks.[10] But this science is still developing. Plastics may be one of the factors leading to chronic illness, but it is not the sole driver. While it is not a reason to panic, it is also not something that should be ignored.

When Plastic Becomes a Problem

Certain everyday habits increase the risk of chemical leaching.
- **Heating plastic**: Microwaving or storing hot food in plastic containers speeds up leaching.
- **Acidic and oily foods**: Tomato chutney or coconut gravies can accelerate plastic breakdown.
- **Old and scratched plastic**: Wear and tear degrades the material and release more compounds.
- **Black plastic containers**: Often made from recycled electronics or contaminated waste, they may contain flame retardants and heavy metals – not what you want your hot curry or dal packed in.

Even products labelled 'BPA-free' can be misleading. Alternatives like BPS and BPF, which are often used in place of BPA, might have similar hormone-disrupting properties. In India, food-grade certifications are loosely regulated, especially for cheap, unbranded plastics sold in local markets.

The Silicone Illusion

Silicone is often marketed as a safer alternative to plastic. It can be, if it is high quality, food grade, and does not smell plasticky when heated. But lower-grade versions often contain fillers and break down over time.

Separating Fact from Fear

Sensational headlines can make plastic seem as harmful as tobacco. Let us analyse this:
- 'You eat a credit card a week': This was an estimate by WWF.[11] The number is debatable, but the concern is valid.
- 'Plastics cause obesity and diabetes': There is some evidence, but the effects are far milder than the impact of food quality and physical activity.

- 'Microplastics are found in the brain': True in some studies, but causality is unclear.

Putting It into Practice

This is not a call to discard all plastic overnight. Start small and be mindful. Never heat food in plastic containers. Use stainless steel, glass, or ceramic for hot, oily, or acidic items. Avoid black plastic takeaway boxes and talk to your local restaurants about safer alternatives. Store spices, grains, and snacks in glass jars or steel containers, and consider replacing non-stick cookware with cast iron or stainless steel once they wear out.

Switching to a steel water bottle, using ceramic mugs, and refusing low-grade plastic from local bazaars are small daily choices that reduce exposure without making you spend too much.

You've Got This

Plastic gave us convenience, but now it is time to use that same ingenuity to choose better options. Instead of chasing a Pinterest-perfect kitchen, build a practical one based on science-backed facts. Understand the risks, select your swaps wisely, and do not fall for eco-fads that are all style and no substance.

6

The Gadget Gamble: Convenience Versus Wellness

Somewhere between villainising the pressure cooker and the air fryer, we have lost the plot. We live in the golden age of kitchen convenience. Look up on Amazon and you will find appliances that give you shortcuts for almost every kitchen chore or claim to help you eat healthier. Food processors with an array of blades you never get around to using, air fryers that promise to 'fry' up everything to a crisp minus the calories, egg boilers, egg poachers, and so on. But somewhere between helpful and harmful lies the real question: which gadgets serve our health, and which serve convenience and speed? News flash: the problem is not the gadget. It is how we use it and how much we let it replace not just the process but the principles of healthy cooking.

Take the microwave. It is often demonised, with myths about radiation and 'killing nutrients' still circulating. But science says otherwise. Microwaving is one of the gentlest cooking methods for preserving water-soluble vitamins like C and B-complex, mainly because it uses less heat and time. The real issue is not the microwave itself but what is inside the pre-packaged, hyper-processed 'microwavable' meals slowly making their way into Indian markets. Now even you will agree, that is not the microwave's fault.

The air fryer is another misunderstood character. It does not fry food in the traditional way. Like an oven on steroids, it circulates hot air to mimic the crispiness of deep frying without using oil. When used wisely for vegetables or healthier baked foods, it can actually boost your health. However, it is easy to fall into the trap of eating more UPFs just because they turn golden and crunchy in 10 minutes. A chicken nugget remains a chicken nugget, whether fried or air-fried.

One of the most common fears in recent years has been that air fryers increase acrylamide formation, a compound formed when starchy foods are cooked at high temperatures, often above 120°C (like frying, roasting, or baking). Acrylamide has been linked to potential cancer risk in animal studies, which understandably raises alarm bells. But there is nuance to this. Acrylamide forms in many cooking methods, including traditional deep frying, baking, and roasting in ovens. The air fryer does not inherently increase acrylamide formation. It simply uses hot circulating air instead of oil. In fact, research shows that air fryers often produce less acrylamide than deep frying, especially when used at lower temperatures and for shorter durations.[12] So, it is not the villain it is often made out to be. The key, as always, is moderation, variety, and mastering how to use your kitchen gadgets wisely. Using your air fryer to make crispy broccoli or sweet potato wedges is very different from air-frying frozen, processed snacks daily.

And what about that rice cooker or Instant Pot? These devices have truly transformed cooking for busy individuals and families. They excel at batch cooking, slow cooking, and pressure cooking – all in one. From homemade yoghurt to preparing healthy lentils or grains in batches with automated start and stop times, these are truly hands-free ways to cook healthy.

What Science Says

Convenience tools, when well-chosen, help people:
- Cook more at home, which is consistently associated with better diet quality.
- Control ingredients, which is vital in managing sodium, sugar, and trans fats.
- Save time and energy, making healthier meals more feasible and cost-effective, especially for working individuals or caregivers.

Research does not support the idea that gadgets like rice cookers, slow cookers, or air fryers are harming our health. In fact, in many Indian homes, the use of a pressure cooker is what makes dal or rajma possible on a busy weekday. Without it, processed alternatives would likely take over. So instead of asking, 'Is this gadget healthy?', a better question might be: 'Does this help me cook fresh, nutrient-dense meals more often?' If yes, it earns a place in your kitchen. If not, it might just be a novelty that takes up counter space and quietly nudges you towards lazy food choices.

The Real Compromise

The real problem is not convenience; it is mindless convenience. The most dangerous gadgets are not the ones on your kitchen counter – they are in your pocket: food delivery apps that turn meals into transactions and provide instant gratification of every food craving.

A well-used air fryer can roast vegetables with hardly any oil. A pressure cooker can help make dals more easily. A good-quality blender can turn soaked millets and dals into a healthy dosa batter or breakfast smoothies on busy mornings. All of these are not just conveniences but also enablers of health.

You've Got This

Ultimately, the smartest kitchen is not the one with the most gadgets. It is the one where technology is thoughtfully integrated and used to support healthy habits, not replace them.

Do not see convenience as the adversary of health. It is a tool, and what really counts is whether it helps you access real food or just makes it easier to avoid it altogether.

7

The Hidden Toxins Lurking in Your Home and How to Send Them Packing

You can track your steps, calories, and sleep with a tap, but not the invisible chemical load in your body. While we obsess over workouts and macros, we may be unaware of toxins from shampoos, sofas, frying pans, and water bottles.

Some people dismiss the idea of 'toxins'. Is not the body designed to detox naturally? It is. But today's chemical overload can overwhelm even our best internal systems. Traces of industrial chemicals and plastic particles now appear in blood, breast milk, and even placentas. This chapter is not meant to scare you but to raise awareness. You do not need to live off-grid or churn your own soap to reduce exposure. You just need to identify where the hidden culprits are and start making smart swaps.

The Sources of Toxins

Indoor air pollution

Many people think of outdoor smog when they hear the term pollution, but indoor air can be just as problematic. In Indian homes, incense sticks, mosquito coils, poorly ventilated kitchens, low-quality synthetic furnishings, and strong-smelling cleaners or air fresheners all contribute to poor indoor air quality. Studies from around the world have shown that indoor air can often be more polluted than outdoor air by a factor of two to five.[13] During and for several hours immediately after certain activities, like paint stripping, levels can reach 1,000 times higher than outdoor levels.

What to do

Keep windows open whenever possible. While it is a popular notion that adding certain indoor plants, like spider plants and snake plants, purifies the air, recent research indicates that you would need an unrealistic number of plants to clean the air as effectively as even one standard air purifier.[14] Research and buy air purifiers for the most frequently used rooms in the house. Use non-toxic cleaning supplies for home cleaning purposes.

Food and packaging

Pesticide residues, plasticisers (like BPA), and preservatives are common in packaged foods. Studies[15] have linked high exposure to endocrine-disrupting chemicals with hormone imbalances, metabolic disorders, and fertility issues. And that 'microwave-safe' plastic container may still be leaching microplastics or phthalates into your leftovers.

What to do

Prioritise fresh, unprocessed food. Store leftovers in glass containers. Wash fruits and vegetables thoroughly, even organic ones. Avoid heating food in plastic, regardless of what the label says.

Household cleaners, detergents, and fragrances

The cleaning aisle of your supermarket is like a chemical theme park. Conventional products often contain ammonia, chlorine bleach, quaternary ammonium compounds, and synthetic fragrances – all ingredients linked to respiratory issues, skin irritation, and hormone disruption. A long-term study found that regular use of household cleaning sprays could damage lungs as much as smoking a pack of cigarettes a day for over 20 years.[16] Scented candles, room sprays, plug-in air fresheners, agarbattis, and even that luxury perfume bottle can emit VOCs (volatile organic compounds) and phthalates. 'Fragrance' on a label can mean hundreds of undisclosed chemicals. In Europe, over 1,300 ingredients are banned in cosmetics. In the US? Just about 11. And India? Let us just say we have some catching up to do.

What to do

Begin with simple steps: switch to a natural deodorant, use fragrance-free lotions, and read labels carefully.

Water contaminants

Most municipal water is treated, but trace amounts of heavy metals, pharmaceutical residues, and microplastics have been detected in tap water across the globe. In India, many cities and towns get borewell water supplied in tankers, where hygiene conditions are questionable. A study[17] reported the presence of microplastics in 81 per cent of global tap water samples.

What to do

Invest in a good water filter. Activated carbon filters can remove chlorine and some chemicals, but RO filters offer broader protection.

Cookware and kitchen surfaces

Non-stick pans may be convenient, but many contain PFAS (polyfluoroalkyl substances). These substances do not break down in the body or the environment and are linked to thyroid problems, immune suppression, and even cancer.

What to do

Ditch scratched non-stick pans. Choose cast iron, stainless steel, or ceramic cookware.

Clothing and home textiles

Clothing labelled 'wrinkle-free' or 'stain-resistant' may be treated with formaldehyde and other chemicals. Flame retardants in mattresses and sofas are also problematic.

What to do

Choose organic cotton or bamboo whenever possible. Wash new clothes before wearing them. And when you get a new mattress or sofa, air it out on the balcony or terrace before using it.

Putting It into Practice

You are the best person to determine your family's exposure to any of the toxins mentioned earlier. Conduct an audit of your home and surroundings, and take steps to replace these with safer alternatives.

You've Got This

You do not have to throw out everything and start from scratch. Make small, consistent choices that lessen your body's burden without sacrificing your sanity. You do not need to live in a bubble. Begin with one change – maybe your water filter or tossing that air freshener. Gradually reduce that toxin load.

Part V

The Hormone Connection

1. How Stress Hormones Quietly Wreck Your Health
2. The Thyroid Puzzle: Beyond the Lab Numbers
3. Testosterone and More: A Man's Guide to Hormonal Health
4. The PCOS Puzzle: One in Five, Still Misunderstood
5. The Hormonal Birth Control Debate
6. Pregnancy and Postpartum: Stripping Away the Myths
7. Perimenopause and Menopause: Navigating the Change

1

How Stress Hormones Quietly Wreck Your Health

We are living in the golden age of wellness – tracking sleep, optimising diets, and perfecting workouts. Yet, despite this biohacking craze, many of us feel worse than ever. The real cause of our stubborn weight gain, broken sleep, and declining energy might be stress hormones quietly causing a biological revolt, one that no celery juice or high-intensity interval training session can control.

The wellness industry has turned 'stress' into a vaguely defined villain, peddling expensive adaptogenic lattes, meditation apps, and retreats that exploit your health anxiety while ignoring deeper hormonal imbalances. Meanwhile, conventional medicine often reduces stress to a psychological issue until it manifests as a physical health condition. Both sides overlook how stress hormones quietly convert daily pressure into genuine health problems.

The Stress Hormone Symphony

The interplay of various hormones in your body is like a symphony orchestra – harmonious and melodious when balanced, and a cacophony when it is not. Your stress response involves much more than just the infamous cortisol. The key players include the following:

- **Cortisol:** It is the primary stress hormone regulated by the hypothalamic-pituitary-adrenal (HPA) axis. Cortisol governs metabolism, controls blood sugar, and, in the acute stage, reduces inflammation to prioritise survival. On the other hand, when chronically elevated, it fuels inflammation, disrupting health. Its secretion follows a circadian rhythm,

peaking in the mornings to energise you and dipping at night for sleep.
- **Adrenaline (epinephrine):** Produced by the adrenal glands (located on top of the kidneys) during acute stress, it increases heart rate, raises blood pressure, and redirects blood flow to muscles for the fight-or-flight response.
- **Noradrenaline (norepinephrine)**: A hormone and neurotransmitter that sharpens focus and alertness, working alongside adrenaline.
- **CRH (corticotropin-releasing hormone):** Released by the hypothalamus, it triggers adrenocorticotropic hormone (ACTH), which then stimulates cortisol. CRH also affects anxiety, appetite, and sleep.

These hormones evolved to handle immediate threats, like escaping a predator. Our stress system, fine-tuned for short, intense survival challenges, is ill-equipped for relentless modern pressures such as endless notifications, financial strain, or work deadlines, which keep it continually activated. Our bodies cannot distinguish a charging lion from a hostile work email; both trigger the same hormonal cascade. Unlike predator encounters, modern stressors linger all day, causing chaos.

What Stress Hormones Actually Do to Your Body

Chronically elevated stress hormones wreak havoc far beyond making you feel 'stressed out'.
- **Immune function**: A *Psychological Bulletin* study found that chronic stress suppresses immunity and increases inflammation, which explains why people tend to get sick more often during stressful times.[1]
- **Cognitive effects**: Research in *Nature Reviews Neuroscience* shows that chronic stress reshapes the brain by enlarging the amygdala (fear centre), while shrinking the prefrontal cortex (decision-making) and hippocampus (memory).[2]
- **Metabolic disruption**: Elevated cortisol increases abdominal fat, leads to insulin resistance, and heightens cravings for calorie-dense foods, undermining even disciplined diets.
- **Cardiovascular impact**: Frequent stress can spike blood pressure, elevate cholesterol levels, and damage arteries, significantly increasing the risk of heart disease.

- **Sleep disruption**: Cortisol and adrenaline oppose melatonin, your sleep hormone. Evening stress makes falling asleep difficult, and sleep deprivation further increases stress hormones.
- **Gut health disruption**: Chronic stress changes gut microbiota and increases intestinal permeability (leaky gut), inflammation, and mood issues. A 2019 *Nature Microbiology* study linked cortisol to microbial imbalances tied to anxiety and digestive problems.[3]

Evidence-Based Strategies to Regulate Stress Hormones

Your stress system responds to targeted interventions:
- **Rhythmic breathing**: Slow breaths (five to six breaths per minute) activate the vagus nerve, helping to shift from stress to relaxation quickly. Try: inhale for four counts, hold for two, exhale for six.
- **Strategic exercise**: Intense workouts temporarily increase cortisol, but regular moderate activity lowers baseline levels. For example, consistent 30 to 40 minutes of moderate exercise per day reduces cortisol.
- **Proper light exposure**: Morning sunlight improves cortisol patterns during the day.
- **Nutrition timing**: Maintaining stable blood sugar helps prevent cortisol spikes. Eating a protein-rich breakfast within an hour of waking stabilises cortisol and insulin levels throughout the day.
- **Social connection**: Physical touch and positive interactions release oxytocin, which counters stress hormones.
- **Psychological reframing**: Viewing stress as an enhancer rather than harm reduces hormonal stress responses. This mindset lowers cortisol and increases DHEA, a growth hormone that balances cortisol.
- **Gut support**: Fermented foods or prebiotics can stabilise gut microbiota disrupted by stress, supporting mood and immunity.

Putting It into Practice

- For acute stress (arguments, deadlines), use quick fixes like deep breathing or a short walk. For chronic stress (work pressure, caregiving), prioritise habits like regular exercise, meditation, and sleep consistency.

- Minimise blood sugar crashes, cut back on inflammatory foods, and limit evening blue light (screens) to prevent further hormonal disruption.

You've Got This

Your stress response is smart and designed to protect you, but only when it works as nature intended. And nature did not intend for stress to be ever present. We have normalised fatigue, anxiety, and inflammation as part of daily life, ignoring the body's signals for a reset. It's time to take charge of the stressors in our lives. Doing so will bring us much closer to true well-being.

2

The Thyroid Puzzle: Beyond the Lab Numbers

If I earned a rupee each time I saw 'Reverse your thyroid' on my Instagram feed, I would never need to work again.

Newsflash: You do not want to *reverse* your thyroid. It is not a disease; it is an organ.

A delicate, butterfly-shaped gland in your neck weighing less than 20 g is now exploited by the wellness industry as its favourite scapegoat.

To take care of your thyroid health, let us explore the middle ground where real science meets genuinely personalised care.

Understanding Thyroid Basics

Your thyroid gland is your body's metabolic command centre. It produces hormones that affect nearly every cell, regulating heart rate, body temperature, energy levels, and how efficiently you burn calories.

The key hormones involved are as follows:
- **T4 (Thyroxine):** The primary hormone made by the thyroid. It is mostly inactive until it is converted into T3.
- **T3 (Triiodothyronine):** The active hormone that fuels metabolism and energy production.
- **TSH (Thyroid-Stimulating Hormone):** Produced by the pituitary gland, it stimulates the thyroid to produce and release thyroid hormones (T3 and T4).

When the thyroid underproduces hormones (hypothyroidism), your system slows down, leading to fatigue, weight gain, dry skin, constipation, cold intolerance, and low mood. When it overproduces hormones (hyperthyroidism), everything speeds up, causing a racing heart (palpitations), anxiety, weight loss, and heat intolerance.

In your basic lab tests, high TSH + low T4 usually indicates hypothyroidism, while low TSH + high T4 usually indicates hyperthyroidism.

Beyond the Standard Testing

Standard thyroid testing for T3, T4, and TSH provides important information, but it is sometimes incomplete for many patients, and additional tests may be needed.
- **Free T3 levels**: Some individuals have normal T4 but find it hard to convert to active T3, causing hypothyroid symptoms despite 'normal' standard tests.
- **Thyroid antibodies**: Hashimoto's thyroiditis, an autoimmune condition that causes hypothyroidism, can be present for years before TSH levels become abnormal. Testing for anti-thyroid peroxidase antibodies can help detect this earlier.
- **Reverse T3**: This inactive form of T3 can increase during stress, illness, or inflammation, effectively blocking the action of regular T3. According to research published in the *Journal of Clinical Endocrinology & Metabolism*, approximately 13 per cent of patients with hypothyroid symptoms have normal TSH levels but could benefit from treatment based on their T3 levels and clinical presentation.[4]

Impact of Food on Thyroid Function

This is a common question among many people with thyroid disorders: What should I eat and avoid? Your diet and lifestyle have a significant impact on your thyroid health, and here are some things to keep in mind.
- **Iodine balance**: Your thyroid needs iodine to produce hormones, but too much can be as problematic as too little. Seafood, dairy, and iodised salt are common sources. Switching from regular iodised salt to more expensive pink or other speciality salts can deprive you of vital iodine and lead to thyroid imbalances.
- **Selenium sufficiency**: This mineral is essential for converting T4 to T3. Brazil nuts, seafood, and eggs are excellent sources.

- **Zinc adequacy**: Zinc deficiency can impair thyroid function and hormone production. Pumpkin seeds, legumes, and shellfish provide this essential mineral.
- **Goitrogens in context**: Certain foods, such as cabbage, broccoli, millets, and soy, contain goitrogens that can interfere with thyroid function, but only when consumed raw and in large amounts. Cooking neutralises most concerns, so do not worry about eating these foods a few times a week in their cooked form.

Be sceptical of 'thyroid diets' promising miraculous results. No single dietary approach works for everyone with thyroid issues. The most evidence-based approach emphasises nutrient adequacy, anti-inflammatory foods, and personalised adjustments based on your response. A diet with adequate protein and healthy fats, including omega-3 fatty acids, is generally considered to support the thyroid.

Some Things to Note About Medication

Medication is typically necessary and beneficial for diagnosed thyroid conditions. However, subtle differences in treatment approaches can significantly impact outcomes.

T4-only medications (like levothyroxine) work well for many patients, but not everyone. Some people do not efficiently convert T4 to active T3.

Take thyroid medication on an empty stomach, consistently at the same time each day, with water. Take it 30 to 60 minutes before eating or drinking tea or coffee. Do not combine it with other supplements like calcium or iron, or with other foods, as this may reduce its absorption.

The 'normal range' for thyroid function is broad. Some patients feel their best at different points within that range. Optimal treatment sometimes means adjusting dosage based on symptoms and lab results.

Putting It into Practice

- If you have classic thyroid symptoms despite 'normal' basic tests, request comprehensive testing, including free T3, free T4, and antibodies.
- Focus on nutrients that support T4 conversion to active T3, such as selenium, zinc, B vitamins, and sufficient protein, while managing stress and prioritising sleep.

- Keep a simple journal of symptoms, energy levels, and medications to identify patterns and optimise your treatment.

You've Got This

Thyroid health exists on a spectrum, not in binary 'normal/abnormal' categories. Your optimal level might differ from population averages. While thyroid dysfunction can cause numerous symptoms, it is rarely the only factor. Sleep quality, stress management, gut health, and other hormonal systems all interact with thyroid function.

Work with doctors who listen to your symptoms and lab results. Managing thyroid health often requires patience and personalised care.

3

Testosterone and More: A Man's Guide to Hormonal Health

Rajeev had not told anyone that he had been feeling his drive fade for months. Not his wife, not his gym buddies, not even his doctor. He chalked it up to stress, work, or just getting older. What he did not realise was that his testosterone was gradually dropping, draining his energy, mood, and muscle mass. Low testosterone is not uncommon. It is rarely discussed though.

Women track their hormones like a second job. Men often joke about women's hormonal swings. Meanwhile, male hormonal health goes unnoticed, undiagnosed, and untreated. The reality is that male hormones also fluctuate. Ignoring them will not solve the problem; addressing it directly could lead to better outcomes.

What Is Going on with Men's Hormones?

Men's biology is a complex system, and testosterone is only one part of it. It drives muscle, libido, energy, mood, and metabolism, but does not work alone. Insulin, cortisol, thyroid hormones, and others constantly interact, and when one malfunctions, the entire system can falter. The surprising part is that these disruptions are affecting men at younger ages and more frequently than ever.

Data paints a stark picture.[5] Average testosterone levels in men today are lower than those of men the same age a few decades ago. This is not just 'ageing'. Chronic stress, reduced sleep, desk-bound jobs, ultra-processed diets, and endocrine-disrupting chemicals in plastics and grooming products are disrupting hormonal balance. The modern world is a hormonal minefield, and men are unknowingly triggering it.

Not Just a Midlife Crisis

Hormonal shifts can start as early as a man's 20s, not just during a midlife crisis. Low testosterone (hypogonadism) does not always signal a 'crisis'. It can develop through subtle, insidious signs such as the following:
- Persistent fatigue or a lack of motivation/energy
- Shrinking muscle mass or stalled strength gains despite lifting weights
- Stubborn belly fat that will not budge
- Fading libido or erectile difficulties
- Mood swings, irritability, or a low-grade sadness
- Slow recovery from workouts or stress

Too many men dismiss these as 'just being tired' or 'part of getting older'. These are red flags worth investigating, especially if they persist.

How Insulin Hijacks Testosterone

Insulin plays a role far beyond diabetes. It is a key player in male hormonal health, similar to its function in women with polycystic ovary syndrome (PCOS). When insulin levels spike due to constant snacking, sugar binges, or a sedentary lifestyle, it can lower testosterone and raise oestrogen. For men, this can show up as:
- Fat accumulating around the belly and chest (the dreaded 'man boobs')
- Relentless cravings, energy crashes, and declining metabolic health
- Sleep apnoea or restless nights

The antidote is building muscle. Resistance training three or four times a week, paired with high-protein meals, can re-sensitise your body to insulin and reset hormonal balance.

Cortisol: The Testosterone Killer

Stress is a hormone wrecker. The constant grind of late-night emails, skipped meals, and doom scrolling floods your system with cortisol, which suppresses testosterone production, disrupts sleep (creating a vicious cycle of low testosterone), adds abdominal fat, and fuels inflammation. It also diminishes sperm production and significantly impacts fertility.

Cortisol is meant for sprints, not marathons. A 24/7 stress lifestyle wears you down over time. Simple daily habits like getting morning sunlight, practising deep breathing, or taking a brisk walk can lower it and protect your hormonal balance.

TRT: Game Changer or Shortcut?

For some men, testosterone replacement therapy (TRT) can be life-changing – boosting energy, mood, libido, muscle mass, and even bone density. In certain cases, it may also reduce the risk of metabolic issues like diabetes. However, it is not a first step or a cure-all. Before considering injections, gels, or patches, eliminate reversible causes such as sleep apnoea, nutrient deficiencies (like low vitamin D or zinc), weak muscle mass, or insulin resistance.

TRT without lifestyle changes (such as strength training, eating nutritious food, and getting better sleep) is like pouring water into a leaky bucket. It might provide a short-term fix, but the underlying problems remain. Additionally, TRT comes with risks like lowered fertility, increased red blood cell count (which can thicken the blood), worsened sleep apnoea, acne, breast enlargement, or potential prostate complications. Men with prostate cancer or heart disease might need to avoid it entirely.

Work with a specialist who can request blood tests to confirm low testosterone, not just rely on symptoms. If TRT is warranted, it must be done under a doctor's supervision, with regular monitoring to adjust doses and catch side effects early.

Putting It into Practice

Hormonal health goes beyond quick fixes or chasing 'alpha' vibes. It is about small, intentional changes that build up over time. Here is your playbook:
- A full panel of blood tests is helpful – total and free testosterone, sex hormone-binding globulin, fasting insulin, HbA1c, vitamin D, and thyroid markers.
- Lift weights three to four times a week. It is the single most effective way to increase testosterone and insulin sensitivity.

Cardio is beneficial, but weight training takes the spotlight here.
- Centre your meals around protein (eggs, meat, fish), fibre (vegetables, whole grains), and healthy fats (avocado, nuts, olive oil). Ditch sugary snacks and ultra-processed carbs.
- Aim for seven to eight hours of sleep each night with a consistent wake-up time. Avoid screens an hour before bed to support melatonin production.

You've Got This

Men's hormones are being hijacked by a world that glorifies stress, screens, and sedentary habits while promoting energy drinks and supplements as solutions. Optimal male health goes beyond aesthetics or performance. It is about energy and resilience that support you through everyday life. If your body has been sending signals, start paying attention and regain control.

4

The PCOS Puzzle: One in Five, Still Misunderstood

Asha, a 30-year-old software engineer, spent years navigating a maze of ineffective 'hormonal healing' supplements promoted by influencers and medical consultations that failed to fully explain her symptoms.

Asha's story is far from unique. Up to one in five Indian women may live with PCOS, yet many face a confusing journey filled with conflicting advice, inconsistent diagnoses, and a lack of clear support. PCOS is a serious hormonal disorder, not a figment of feminine imagination, and it requires compassion and science-backed care to address its complexities.

Understanding PCOS Beyond the Name

'Polycystic ovary syndrome' is a misleading name. You can have PCOS without any ovarian cysts, and cysts do not always mean PCOS.

At its core, PCOS is a hormonal disorder that affects metabolism, menstrual cycles, skin, fertility, and even mental health.

Doctors diagnose it using the Rotterdam criteria, which require two out of three signs: irregular or absent periods, elevated male hormones (detected through blood tests or symptoms like acne, excess hair growth, or hair loss), or ovaries that appear 'polycystic' on an ultrasound. However, these criteria do not capture the whole picture.

PCOS varies widely. Some women experience ovulation problems; others have insulin resistance or visible symptoms like hirsutism (excess hair). India's urban lifestyle, with late nights, processed foods, stress, and pollution, can worsen these hormonal imbalances, especially for those with a genetic predisposition.

Symptoms often start in adolescence with irregular periods or acne and may continue into the reproductive years and beyond, sometimes shifting in perimenopause. While typically diagnosed early, PCOS can be identified later if symptoms like insulin resistance emerge or if earlier signs were missed.

The Insulin Connection

PCOS is closely linked to insulin resistance, a connection often overlooked. About 70 per cent of women with PCOS have insulin resistance. It means your cells do not respond properly to insulin, so your body produces more of it. That leads to the following:
- More androgens (causing acne and facial hair)
- Disrupted ovulation
- Trouble losing weight (no, you are not lazy)
- Sugar cravings and 'hangry' spells
- Higher risk of type 2 diabetes

You do not even have to be overweight to have insulin resistance. And when you improve insulin sensitivity through food, movement, and sleep, things start to fall into place. A 2020 study by *The Lancet* found that even a modest 5–10 per cent weight loss (if necessary) can restore ovulation by improving insulin function, not just by reducing weight.[6]

Beyond Birth Control Pills and Metformin

Conventional treatments often include the following:
- Birth control pills to regulate periods
- Metformin to address insulin resistance

While these can manage symptoms, they do not address root causes and may not be suitable for everyone. A sustainable, evidence-based approach includes the following:
- **Anti-inflammatory diet**: Emphasise whole foods like vegetables, lentils, whole grains, seeds, and healthy fats. Limit UPFs. No significant clinical trials support gluten-free diets as

better for PCOS management, so avoid restrictive trends unless medically necessary.
- **Strength over cardio**: Gentle strength training and walking are more effective than high-intensity workouts, which can elevate cortisol levels and worsen hormonal imbalances.
- **Sleep and light exposure**: Maintaining regular sleep schedules and getting morning sunlight helps support hormonal rhythms.
- **Smart supplements**: Inositol (myo- and D-chiro-inositol in a 40:1 ratio) can improve insulin sensitivity and promote ovulation with fewer side effects than metformin. Consult your doctor before starting.

What About Fertility?

PCOS is a leading cause of infertility, but many women can conceive with the right approach. A tailored plan often includes the following:
- Improving insulin sensitivity
- Tracking ovulation with apps, basal body temperature, or LH strips
- Timing intercourse or insemination
- Medications like letrozole or clomiphene, as prescribed by a gynaecologist

Balancing hormones restores fertility for many. Personalisation is key, as no one plan fits all.

Putting It into Practice

- **Seek comprehensive testing**: Test insulin, glucose, and inflammatory markers to identify the cause of PCOS.
- **Prioritise insulin sensitivity**: Eat regular meals containing protein, fibre, and healthy fats, and incorporate strength training while maintaining a consistent sleep routine.
- **Track patterns**: Log cycles to identify triggers and responses, as PCOS varies widely.

You've Got This

PCOS is a metabolic disorder influenced by lifestyle and environment, intersecting with genetic predispositions. Modern challenges like pesticide-laden foods, late-night screen use, and chronic stress increase its effects. Genuine PCOS care management involves moving away from quick fixes and building hormonal resilience through informed nutrition, adequate rest, activity, and medical support.

5

The Hormonal Birth Control Debate

The birth control pill, taken daily by millions of women around the world, remains a paradox: a symbol of freedom and a source of controversy. Depending on whom you ask, it is either a feminist victory or a hormone disruptor. The truth is that it is both, and that is where things become complicated.

In a world where young women are handed pills like laddoos at a wedding, explanations are often lacking. Teens are prescribed the pill for acne, irregular periods, or severe cramps, often before they understand their own cycles. Prescriptions are given without explaining how the pill affects hormones or what alternatives are available. Not just as a contraceptive, it becomes a catch-all for any menstrual issue, which is problematic when it masks underlying issues like PCOS or endometriosis.

There is no doubt that the pill's ability to prevent pregnancy is a game-changer. By giving women control over when to have kids, it has opened doors to education, careers, and financial independence. Economists have even linked it to a rise in women joining the workforce and boosting economic growth. The pill is a marvel of medical progress, but it is also not without its fine print.

How the Pill Works

The most common birth control pills are made from synthetic oestrogen and progestin (a lab-made version of progesterone). These hormones work in three ways to prevent pregnancy: they stop ovulation, thicken cervical mucus to block sperm, and thin the uterine lining to make it difficult for a fertilised egg to implant. In short, they override your body's natural hormonal cycle, replacing it with a predictable, lab-crafted cycle that feels anything but natural.

For many, this offers benefits. Periods become lighter and more regular. Acne clears up. Endometriosis pain eases. PMS stops feeling like an emotional freefall. For women with PCOS or other hormonal imbalances, the pill can be a lifeline, controlling symptoms like unwanted hair growth or erratic cycles. However, there is no hiding that this could be a bandage rather than a lasting, true solution for underlying issues.

Pills are not the only option for contraception. Patches, vaginal rings, hormonal IUDs, and injections offer similar effectiveness but with different delivery methods. A weekly patch or a five-year IUD might seem more convenient than taking a daily pill, but each has its own fine print, from skin irritation to mood changes. Choose wisely.

What Is the Trade-Off?

While hormonal birth control can offer stability, it may also suppress the natural hormonal ebbs and flows that are part of your body's design. Some women report mood changes, decreased libido, weight gain, or feeling emotionally flat while on the pill, whereas others do not experience these symptoms.

Emerging research also indicates that the pill may slightly raise the risk of blood clots, stroke, and breast cancer in some women, especially those who smoke or are over 35.[7] On the other hand, long-term use is associated with a reduced risk of ovarian and endometrial cancers.

There is also growing interest in how hormonal contraceptives impact the gut microbiome and nutrient absorption (like magnesium and B vitamins). These areas are still being studied, but they suggest the pill's effects extend beyond just the reproductive system.

What About Non-Hormonal Alternatives?

Some people rely on natural methods which involve tracking temperature, cervical mucus, and cycle patterns to predict fertile windows. There are apps on smartphones that help identify the fertile window. When practised perfectly, these methods can be up to 99 per cent effective. Still, with typical use, its effectiveness drops to about 76–88 per cent, meaning roughly one in four to one in eight women using only this method may become pregnant within a year.

Non-hormonal options provide alternatives worth considering:
- The copper IUD is over 99 per cent effective, hormone-free, and can last up to 10 years. It works by creating a sperm-repelling environment in the uterus but may cause heavier periods, especially in the beginning.
- Barrier methods such as condoms (82–98 per cent effective depending on use), vaginal sponges, diaphragms, and cervical caps (the latter two are less popular in India) provide hormone-free protection but require consistent and correct use with each sexual encounter.

Each option has its own mix of effectiveness, convenience, and potential side effects. The 'best' method varies from woman to woman.

Finding What Works for You

The oral contraceptive pill is not entirely harmful, but it is not harmless either. Like any powerful medication, it has effects beyond its main purpose. For some, the benefits outweigh the risks. For others, they do not.

What matters most is that women receive the complete picture. Hormonal birth control can be offered when necessary, but it should not be given as a one-size-fits-all solution for every hormonal problem. Women should be encouraged to ask questions like: why am I taking this? Is it making me feel better? What are my alternatives?

Some women feel like their best selves on the pill. Others feel like strangers in their own bodies. Both experiences are valid. There's no one-size-fits-all approach to hormones, and that's the most important thing to remember.

Putting It into Practice

- If you are on the pill and feeling good, that is great. Stay informed and in touch with your gynaecologist.
- If you are experiencing mood swings, brain fog, or other symptoms, consult your doctor.
- Consider a complete hormonal workup before starting or switching methods.

- Nutrient support (like magnesium, B-complex, and zinc) can help compensate for some pill-related depletions.

You've Got This

When the discourse is full of noise, conflicting advice, and pharmaceutical marketing, the smartest move is to stay curious and aware. Hormonal birth control is neither the enemy nor the saviour of your health; it is simply a tool. And tools are most effective when you know exactly how to use them. You do not need to fear the pill, nor do you need to blindly trust it. Instead, you should understand your body well enough to decide what is right for you.

6

Pregnancy and Postpartum: Stripping Away the Myths

This topic warrants its own book. Pregnancy and postpartum care influence nearly every facet of women's physical, emotional, nutritional, and social health. In India, these experiences are often surrounded by tradition, taboos, and endless advice from all parts of the family (and now, even social media). While some of that wisdom is timeless, much of it needs to be reconsidered and updated. In this chapter, we will focus on debunking myths and providing you with science-backed, compassionate guidance for what is often one of the most transformative and vulnerable times in a woman's life.

Nutrition and Exercise During Pregnancy

Myth: you are eating for two.
Truth: you are eating for one person who happens to be growing another.

Pregnancy increases nutritional needs, but not significantly. Most women require only an additional 300–500 calories per day, mainly during the second and third trimesters. What is more important is nutrient density, not just the total quantity. Key nutrients include iron, calcium, protein, choline, folate, and omega-3 fatty acids. In Indian diets, this can include a mix of ragi, leafy greens, dal, eggs or paneer, sesame seeds, flaxseed chutney, fish, chicken, and more.

You do not have to stop exercising unless your doctor advises you to for a specific reason. In fact, regular movement during pregnancy can improve mood, digestion, sleep, and even labour outcomes. Walking, prenatal yoga, and gentle strength training are safe for most women. If you were active before pregnancy, you can usually keep it up with some modifications. Always listen to your body. Pain, dizziness, or shortness of breath are signals to stop and consult your doctor.

Postpartum Recovery: Physical and Emotional

What happens after birth is often overlooked in conversations, but this stage is equally important. It is rightfully called the fourth trimester. Your uterus is shrinking, hormones are recalibrating, and you might be dealing with stitches, haemorrhoids, leaking breasts, and a body that does not feel like your own. It takes time to return to normal.

In many Indian homes, the 40-day confinement period is treated as sacred and rightly so. However, it does not mean total passivity or being fed three to four ghee- and sugar-laden laddoos daily. What is needed is nourishing food, gentle movement (like walking), plenty of rest, and pelvic floor care.

Pelvic physiotherapy, especially after vaginal delivery, is vital but rarely discussed. It helps recover from prolapse, incontinence, and core dysfunction. These are fixable problems.

The Invisible Cloak of Postpartum Depression

Myth: You should be glowing with happiness after your baby arrives. Truth: You might be crying for no reason, feel rage, or feel nothing at all, and that is valid.

Postpartum depression (PPD) affects around one in seven women globally. It can present as anxiety, numbness, guilt, panic, or intrusive thoughts. In India, PPD often goes unrecognised because of shame, social expectations from new mothers, and a lack of support.

Therapy, community support, and, in some cases, medication can help with PDD. Ignoring or labelling it as 'baby blues' can have long-term consequences for both mother and child.

Untreated maternal mental health conditions can impact infant development, bonding, and future mental health. Just as we prioritise vaccines and nutrition, we must also prioritise maternal mental health. If you or someone you love appears to be struggling after giving birth, ask questions, listen, and offer support without judgement.

The Role of Family and Support Systems

In Indian households, new mothers are celebrated as queens but are often left without a safety net. True support goes beyond verbal reassurances of 'just rest' while the chores pile up. It means dads washing bottles, grandparents rocking the baby to sleep, siblings running errands, or anyone simply asking, 'How are you holding up?' Every family member has a role that is more than just attending the naming ceremony.

Some traditions, though wrapped in love, are outdated. Confining a mother indoors for weeks, banning baths, or force-feeding ghee- and sugar-laden sweets to 'rebuild strength' can be more harmful than helpful. Science shows that fresh air and balanced meals beat isolation and sugar overload. Choose what nourishes your body and soul – maybe warm turmeric milk, not 40 days of house arrest – and let go of what does not. Your postpartum journey, your rules.

Breastfeeding: Facts Versus Myths

Myth: If you do not produce milk immediately, you have failed.
Truth: Colostrum (the early milk) appears in small amounts but is potent and perfect.

Milk supply increases over time with stimulation and support. India has high breastfeeding initiation rates, but continued exclusive breastfeeding drops off sharply after the first month, often due to misinformation, poor latching by the baby, or the need to return to work soon after delivery.

Here are some truths:
- Breastfeeding might not feel instinctive. It is a learned skill. Qualified lactation consultants or your doctor can advise you.
- Supplementing with formula is not shameful. Some babies need more, and some mothers face challenges.
- Pumping milk and storing it in the fridge is another way to ensure the baby can access breast milk when the mom is away.

You've Got This

Pregnancy and postpartum are intense, transformative journeys. Your body reshapes, your identity shifts, and your relationships transform under new expectations. The exhaustion, joy, overwhelming emotions – it is all real.

Eliminate the pressure to snap back into skinny jeans or be the perfect, self-sacrificing mom. Instead, let us demand genuine care – a family and community that shows up and science that respects your body's truth. Whether you are a new mom, expecting, or supporting someone through it, reshape the narrative with heart and humanity. And never hesitate to ask for the help you deserve.

7

Perimenopause and Menopause: Navigating the Change

Society has got it all wrong. Menopause is not the end of your prime. It is a midlife revolution, reshaping your body and mind for a bold new chapter. Perimenopause, the years of hormonal ups and downs before your periods stop, and menopause, when cycles end (typically in your late 40s to early 50s), unleash a wave of changes like hot flashes, mood swings, and more. For women worldwide, juggling family, work, and societal pressures, these shifts can hit hard. Armed with science-backed tools like balanced diets, structured movement, and exercise, you can navigate this transition with strength, clarity, and a whole lot of grit.

So What Happens Exactly?

Perimenopause, often kicking off in your 40s, causes oestrogen and progesterone levels to fluctuate wildly. This hormonal chaos results in irregular periods, hot flashes, night sweats, and sleep disruptions.

Menopause is marked by 12 months without a period, typically in your late 40s to early 50s. But it is not just your ovaries saying goodbye. Oestrogen shapes mood, memory, and temperature regulation, so its decline can disrupt your internal thermostat and cause emotional swings like a pendulum gone rogue.

A 2018 study in *Menopause* found that cognitive behavioural therapy (CBT) reduced the severity of hot flashes and night sweats by 30 per cent compared to standard care.[8] Your brain's perception of these symptoms influences how intense they feel. Rewiring how you interpret these signals can help you decrease the heat, both physically and mentally.

Menopause is not a flaw in human biology but an evolutionary feature. The grandmother hypothesis proposes that women evolved to live long after their reproductive years to support their families, increase the survival chances of grandchildren, and pass down wisdom. This view presents menopause as a strategic advantage, not a weakness.

Taming the Symptoms

While hot flashes come across as its brand ambassador, menopause comes with many more symptoms.

- **Hot flashes and night sweats**: These sudden heat surges can interrupt sleep and daily routines. Cooling methods like sipping cold water, wearing breathable, loose cotton kurtas or kaftans, or practising paced breathing can help. Yoga, rooted in Indian tradition, lowers hot flash frequency by calming the nervous system. Learn specific asanas or pranayamas from a teacher.
- **Mood swings**: Oestrogen dips can make you feel like you are starring in an emotional soap opera. Mindfulness meditation steadies the mind. Regular chats with friends or a therapist can also keep you grounded.
- **Sleep disruptions**: Poor sleep worsens mood swings and fatigue. Maintaining a consistent bedtime routine (replace late-night WhatsApp scrolling with chamomile tea) and keeping a cool, dark bedroom can improve rest.
- **Cognitive fog**: Struggling to recall names or concentrate? Oestrogen supports brain function, so its decline can cloud cognition. Mental exercises like Sudoku or learning a new skill (try a salsa class) help keep your brain sharp.

Should You Consider HRT?

Hormone replacement therapy (HRT), once demonised, is making a scientific comeback. When used appropriately, HRT can reduce hot flashes, maintain bone density, improve mood symptoms, and potentially protect heart health if started at the right time. The Women's Health Initiative in 2002 sparked widespread fear over breast cancer risks.[9] However, new data indicate that for most healthy women under 60, the benefits far outweigh the risks when

HRT is tailored and closely monitored. There are multiple types of HRT, such as oestrogen-only, combined (with progesterone), and even body-identical hormones.

India still has progress to make in awareness around HRT, but it is valuable to have an open, nuanced conversation with your gynaecologist.

Your Perimenopause and Menopause Toolkit

Your daily habits form the scaffolding for this midlife rebuild. Some simple practices can help fortify your foundation:

- **Movement**: Exercise is not just for fitness. It also balances hormones. The *Journal of Mid-Life Health Review* shows moderate activity, like brisk walking or yoga, reduces menopausal symptoms.[10] Aim for 30 minutes, 5 days a week. Bonus: it boosts mood and sleep.

  Lifting weights or using resistance bands builds muscle and increases bone density, helping to counteract menopause-related bone loss. Start with guidance from a trainer and do not hesitate to progressively lift heavier weights, doing compound exercises like squats, deadlifts, bench presses, and shoulder presses, among others.
- **Nutrition**: Oestrogen's decline increases risks for osteoporosis and heart disease. Support your body with the following:
  (i) **Calcium and Vitamin D:** Dairy, ragi, sesame seeds, and 10 to 15 minutes of morning sunlight or a vitamin D supplement
  (ii) **Anti-inflammatory foods:** Turmeric, ginger, pomegranate, kiwi, nuts, and omega-3s from fish or flaxseeds protect your brain and joints.
  (iii) **Protein:** You may need more now than in your 30s to preserve muscle and metabolism. Aim for 1–1.5 g/kg of body weight per day.
- **Stress management**: Chronic stress spikes cortisol, worsening hot flashes and mood swings. Doing daily pranayama (breathing exercises) or walking in the park can reduce stress. A calm mind results in a calm body.
- **Connection**: Do not underestimate the healing power of friendship. Loneliness affects health (and lifespan) more than

smoking. Whether it is tea with your neighbour or a Sunday call with cousins, stay connected.

Putting It into Practice

There is no single fix for menopause; it requires a team effort. Combine these strategies for the best results:
- **Physical tools**: A combination of walking, strength training, yoga, and any other enjoyable movements to maintain strength and flexibility.
- **Mental strategies**: Cognitive behavioural therapy, mindfulness, or journalling to manage emotional and cognitive shifts.
- **Lifestyle upgrades**: Prioritise sleep, eat nutrient-dense foods, and nurture friendships.

Recommended reading
- *The Menopause Manifesto* by Dr Jen Gunter: A no-nonsense guide to understanding and managing menopause with science and humour.

You've Got This

Do not look at menopause as a decline. Instead, treat it as an opportunity to rebuild yourself. The commoditisation of menopause might scare you into taking hormone pills, special diets, or potions. With movement, nutrition, mental strategies, and community, you can turn this phase into a positive and enriching experience.

Part VI

Sleep: The Missing Superpower

1. Mastering Rest: The Secrets to Deep, Restorative Sleep
2. The Battle Between Modern Life and Sleep
3. Are You Socially Jetlagged?
4. Snoring: A Red Flag for Your Health
5. Sleep and Mental Health: A Two-Way Street

1

Mastering Rest: The Secrets to Deep, Restorative Sleep

It's a commonly heard notion that, to go to sleep, you have to pretend to be asleep until you actually fall asleep.

Imagine this: a dark, quiet room at the ideal temperature. Fresh sheets topped with a pillow that supports your head and neck perfectly. How wonderful it would be to slip under the covers and enjoy a restful, uninterrupted sleep for seven to eight hours.

We spend a third of our lives sleeping – or trying to sleep. But in a world that glorifies overwork, sleep has become somewhat of an embarrassment. No one posts their full eight hours of sleep on LinkedIn. Instead, sleeplessness is worn like a badge – proof that you are busy, important, indispensable.

In this chapter, we will reclaim what should never have been lost: the right to rest deeply and unapologetically.

What Happens When We Sleep?

Sleep is much more than just 'resting'. It is a complex biological process essential for physical, mental, and emotional health. Our sleep occurs in cycles between two primary types: REM (rapid eye movement) and NREM (non-rapid eye movement) sleep.

During NREM sleep, especially the deeper stages, the body enters repair mode. Muscles recover, tissues grow, immune function strengthens, and the brain consolidates memories. It is somewhat like backing up your hard drive: short-term memories are stored as long-term ones.

REM sleep, on the other hand, is when your brain becomes more active. This is when you dream. It is during REM that the brain processes the day's experiences, emotions, and learning – stitching together the story of your life. According to neuroscientist Matthew

Walker, author of *Why We Sleep*, if you do not sleep the night after learning something new, you miss the window to consolidate those memories. This highlights how important sleep is for students.

Walker describes deep NREM sleep as 'one of the most epic displays of neural collaboration that we know of'.[1] Thousands of neurons fire together in harmony, helping the brain reset and prepare for the next day.

The High Cost of Skimping on Sleep

Modern life makes sleep difficult. With late-night screen time, erratic schedules, and round-the-clock work emails and pings, it is no wonder many of us struggle to get quality sleep. Chronic sleep deprivation, which can occur even from losing just one to two hours a night over time, can impair memory, cognitive function, emotional control, and immunity.

Poor sleep has been linked to everything from weight gain and diabetes to heart disease and even cancer. A week of moderately reduced sleep can disrupt blood sugar levels just as much as it would in someone with pre-diabetes. For those in creative or high-performance fields, this is crucial: sleep fuels insight, decision-making, and emotional resilience. Do we need more reasons to give deep sleep the importance it deserves?

Eleven Evidence-Backed Tips for Better Sleep

Fortunately, there is a lot we can do to reclaim restful sleep. These research-backed habits can help reset your natural rhythms:

- **Get morning sunlight**: Spending at least 30 minutes in sunlight during the day helps regulate your circadian rhythm and signals to your brain that it is time to wake up.
- **Stick to a consistent schedule**: Go to bed and wake up at the same time every day, even on weekends. Consistency strengthens your internal body clock.
- **Skip late naps**: Napping after 3 p.m. can disrupt nighttime sleep. If you need to nap, keep it under 30 minutes and before mid-afternoon.
- **Avoid stimulants**: Refrain from caffeine and nicotine in the hours before bedtime. These can delay sleep onset and lower sleep quality.

- **Time your workouts**: Finish exercise at least three to four hours before bedtime. While movement supports good sleep, vigorous workouts too late in the day can be stimulating.
- **Limit alcohol**: While a nightcap may help you fall asleep, it disrupts sleep architecture, particularly REM sleep, leaving you groggy the next day.
- **Create a wind-down routine**: Dim the lights, turn off screens, read a book, or listen to calming music. Let your body know it is time to wind down.
- **Make your bedroom a sanctuary**: Keep it cool, dark, and quiet. Invest in quality bedding and remove electronic devices that emit blue light.
- **Watch what you eat**: Stay away from heavy meals and sugar near bedtime. If you are hungry, a light snack like a banana or warm milk can help.
- **Manage stress**: Journalling, meditation, and deep breathing exercises can help calm a racing mind before bed.
- **Limit screen time before bed**: Blue light from phones and laptops suppresses melatonin, the sleep hormone. Try switching to night mode or going screen-free an hour before bed.

Sleep and Hustle Culture

During our peak career years, work is often the biggest thief of sleep. Tight deadlines, endless conference calls, and a culture that glorifies late nights can all disrupt our circadian rhythm. But there are ways to course-correct.

Start with work hygiene. Avoid scheduling meetings after work hours or setting unrealistic deadlines that lead to late-night catch-ups. Discourage glorifying burning the midnight Wi-Fi. Instead, establish healthy boundaries and prioritise sleep. Help build a workplace culture where rest is viewed as a productivity tool, not a weakness.

Simple changes at the workplace can make a big difference. Optimising workspace lighting to mirror natural light helps regulate the body's internal clock. Consider creating a dedicated nap zone for short power naps, an evidence-based practice that boosts alertness and creativity.

Putting It into Practice

Starting tonight, pick one change from the earlier-mentioned list, such as dimming lights an hour before bed or skipping that evening scroll. Stick with it for the next seven days. Small changes add up to significant results.

Recommended reading

- *Why We Sleep: Unlocking the Power of Sleep and Dreams* by Matthew Walker

You've Got This

Sleep is an active process where the body and mind engage in vital restoration. When we learn to prioritise sleep, we do not just feel better, we function better. Rest is not indulgence; it is simply honouring our body's most fundamental need.

2

The Battle Between Modern Life and Sleep

Ranjani was wide awake at midnight, alert but exhausted. She had promised herself just 10 minutes to unwind after dinner, but that turned into two hours of flicking through vegan recipe reels and skincare hacks. When she finally dragged herself to bed, she could not sleep. Her body was wired, her brain buzzing. Two hours of 'relaxation' had given her a solid dose of screen-induced insomnia.

Sounds familiar? It is not your fault. We live in a world that is rigged against rest. One of the most silent casualties of modern living is deep, restorative sleep. The tools we use for relaxation – Netflix, social media, late-night snacks, entertainment on our phones – are not helping us wind down. They are stimulating us to exhaustion.

The Blue Light Business

Let us begin with blue light, the short-wavelength light emitted by screens. Blue light in the natural world is beneficial. It signals your body that it is morning and time to wake up. However, when the same signal reaches your eyes at 11 p.m. from a phone screen, it disrupts your internal clock, suppresses melatonin (the hormone responsible for sleep), and shifts your body into alert mode. This can delay sleep onset, reduce sleep quality, and interfere with your natural circadian rhythm.

It is not just your phone. Televisions, tablets, and laptops, especially when used close to bedtime, have a cumulative effect. And yes, blue light filter mode helps a bit, but it does not counteract the stimulation and dopamine hits from endless scrolling or late-night WhatsApp group chats with friends.

The Binge Culture

Even if you are not scrolling, there is a good chance you are bingeing – whether it is a show, YouTube videos, or that bag of chips. Our brains crave predictable dopamine hits, and streaming platforms have perfected the art of keeping us hooked with autoplay, cliffhangers, and infinite scroll.

But bingeing has consequences. Overeating late at night not only impairs digestion and contributes to weight gain but also disrupts your body's internal cues for rest. Your body should be in parasympathetic mode at night, ready for repair, not processing an ice cream or decoding a crime-thriller plot.

Even the good old habit of reading before bed can backfire if the content is too intense or if you are on an e-reader with a bright screen. It is all about overstimulation. Our brains are simply not designed to stay in fight-or-flight mode until midnight.

Modern Life Has Killed the Wind-Down

The final piece of this puzzle is the lack of boundaries in modern life. Work emails at 9 p.m., 'urgent' client calls right before bed, the group chat that comes alive at 10 p.m. – our brains never truly shut down because we do not give them permission to.

Sleep needs a winding-down process, a buffer zone between the chaos of the day and the calm of the night. Without it, we carry the day into our dreams, if we even manage to sleep at all.

The Fallout

Chronic sleep deprivation is not just about feeling tired. It affects everything – your blood sugar control, appetite regulation, immune function, memory, mood, and even skin health. Ironically, the more tired you are, the more likely you are to reach for quick dopamine fixes like sugar, caffeine, or another episode of a series, creating a vicious cycle that is hard to break.

Putting It into Practice

Here is your sleep repair toolkit:
- **Set a sleep boundary**: Choose a non-negotiable bedtime and work backwards to include at least 30–60 minutes of wind-down time.

- **Screen curfew**: Turn off devices at least 60 to 90 minutes before bed. Read a physical book, journal, or simply lie in the dark and breathe.
- **Protect your circadian rhythm**: Get bright light exposure during the day and keep evenings dim. If possible, aim for outdoor light first thing in the morning.
- **Close the kitchen early**: Aim to finish dinner at least two to three hours before bedtime so your body can focus on sleep, not digestion.
- **No phones near the bed**: Buy an old-fashioned alarm clock. Your phone should sleep in another room.
- **Create rituals**: A cup of herbal tea, stretching, or gratitude journalling signals your body that sleep is coming.

You've Got This

You do not have to live like a monk to get good sleep, but you do need to draw a line somewhere. Sleep is a basic need for good health. It influences every health goal you have ever pursued, whether it is fat loss, better mood, sharper focus, or balanced hormones.

Reclaim your sleep, and everything else begins to fall into place.

3

Are You Socially Jetlagged?

Every Friday night, Akash, a digital agency executive, relaxes with a few hours of binge-watching. Saturday and Sunday mornings are protected times when he sleeps without guilt. By Monday, he feels groggy, irritable, and has trouble focusing. He attributes it to a 'bad Monday' or simply not being a morning person. However, what Akash is experiencing is not a personality flaw or a productivity issue. It is a modern epidemic called *social jetlag*.

And it is quietly dismantling health and performance worldwide, one well-intentioned weekend at a time.

What Is Social Jetlag?

Social jetlag is the discrepancy between biological time, determined by our internal body clock, and social time, mainly dictated by social obligations such as school, work, or play. Unlike traditional jet lag caused by travel, social jetlag is self-imposed, caused by staying up late and sleeping in on weekends, only to shift back to early mornings during the week. Think of it as a recurring mini jet lag that resets every Monday. The greater the gap between your weekday and weekend sleep schedules, the more your internal clock struggles to adjust. Research shows that more than one hour of difference between your weekday and weekend sleep has a significant impact.[2] Most people go beyond that benchmark quite routinely.

Why It Matters

Our body does not know the difference between a weekday and a weekend (and free days). Any disruption in the schedule adds up over the weeks and months. This repeated circadian disruption does not just lead to groggy mornings. Research links

social jetlag to a variety of adverse health outcomes, including the following[3]:
- Increased risk of obesity, type 2 diabetes, and insulin resistance
- Higher rates of depression, anxiety, and irritability
- Reduced attention span, slower reaction times, and impaired memory
- Elevated blood pressure and increased risk of heart disease
- Additionally, chronic social jetlag can weaken the immune system, impair recovery from workouts, and reduce overall quality of life

The Sleep–Performance Connection

Sleep consistency is crucial for optimal performance, both physical and cognitive. Athletes who maintain regular sleep schedules tend to have better reaction times, endurance, and injury recovery.[4] In the workplace, irregular sleep can lead to decreased productivity, more mistakes, and poor decision-making. Your brain and body function best when your circadian rhythm aligns with your environment. When that rhythm constantly shifts due to social jetlag, it is like asking your body to operate in a different time zone every week.

Who Is Most at Risk?

Social jetlag affects all age groups, but adolescents and young adults are especially vulnerable because of their natural tendency to sleep and wake up late. Early school or work schedules during the week lead them to accumulate significant sleep debt, which they try to repay on weekends or holidays, worsening the cycle. Shift workers and frequent travellers also face severe forms of social jetlag. Even a consistent 90-minute weekend delay can have noticeable effects on health.

How to Minimise Social Jetlag?

Here are some ways to reduce the effects of social jetlag:
- Stick to a consistent sleep schedule. Try to go to bed and wake up at about the same time every day, including weekends. A variation of no more than an hour is ideal.

- Prioritise sleep during the week. Do not depend on weekends to catch up. Make sleep a priority on weekdays. About seven to nine hours of sleep per night is ideal for most adults.
- Use light wisely. Morning sunlight helps anchor your circadian rhythm. Open your curtains or take a short walk outside soon after waking.
- Limit exposure to evening light. Blue light from screens can delay melatonin production. Try dimming lights and avoiding devices at least an hour before bed.
- Avoid oversleeping. While it is tempting, sleeping until noon disrupts your sleep–wake cycle. If you are tired, consider a short nap (20 to 30 minutes) instead.
- Be mindful of social and work commitments. Plan late-night outings sparingly and try to finish them earlier, whenever possible, to avoid disrupting your sleep schedule.

Putting It into Practice

Managing social jetlag is about creating an overall lifestyle that promotes healthy rest. You can begin with these simple changes:
- Avoid caffeine at least six hours before bed.
- Engage in relaxing activities like reading or stretching to cue your body for sleep.
- Regular physical activity and balanced nutrition support more stable energy rhythms and better sleep quality.

You've Got This

In a culture of constant activity and stimulation, sleep is often sacrificed for socialising, entertainment, or work. But this weekly misalignment has consequences. Social jetlag may seem harmless, but over time, it gradually affects your health, mood, and performance.

Protect your internal clock and provide your body with the stability it needs to thrive.

4

Snoring: A Red Flag for Your Health

In Indian cinema, snoring is often used for comedic relief. It is the soundtrack of a father-in-law dozing off mid-conversation or a clumsy uncle passed out after a wedding feast. And for decades, we have laughed along.

But when mainstream Tamil cinema makes a movie like *Good Night*, focused on the emotional and social impact of loud snoring and sleep apnoea, you know the issue has moved from a punchline to a central theme. It has transformed from a harmless quirk to a health hazard.

The Mechanics Behind Snoring

Snoring happens when air cannot flow easily through your airway during sleep. As you breathe, the relaxed tissues in your throat vibrate, producing the snoring sound. But why does this occur? Common causes include the following:

- Excess weight around the neck and throat
- Anatomical features like a narrow airway or a deviated nasal septum
- Alcohol consumption before bed, which over-relaxes the throat muscles
- Nasal congestion caused by allergies or sinus issues
- Age-related loss of muscle tone
- Sleeping position (particularly sleeping on your back)

When snoring becomes severe or is accompanied by pauses in breathing followed by gasping or choking, it may indicate obstructive sleep apnoea (OSA), a serious sleep disorder that requires medical attention.

While occasional snoring can be harmless (after a long day, a heavy meal, or a blocked nose from a common cold), chronic snoring is rarely just snoring. It can be a warning sign of OSA, where the airway repeatedly gets blocked during sleep, causing breathing to stop and start. You might not even realise this is happening, but your body does. Each time breathing stops, even for a few seconds, your oxygen levels drop and your brain jolts awake slightly to restore airflow. This results in fragmented sleep, and you wake up tired despite spending seven to eight hours in bed.

Who Is at Risk?

Although snoring is often associated with older men or those with higher body weight, it is not limited to them. Women can also develop sleep apnoea, especially post-menopause. Children who snore regularly should be checked, especially if they appear sleepy or irritable during the day.

Factors like genetics, neck circumference, alcohol intake, and even sleeping posture can all contribute. And yes, thin people snore too. While excess body weight increases the risk, it is not the only factor.

The Silent Damage

When snoring is part of a larger sleep apnoea pattern, it affects your body in many ways. Untreated sleep apnoea goes beyond just sleep issues. Poor concentration, memory lapses, constant fatigue, irritability, and mood swings are just the start. Over time, the condition increases the risk of high blood pressure, insulin resistance, diabetes, stroke, and even heart disease. And let us not forget the impact on relationships. Many couples end up sleeping in separate rooms simply because one partner's snoring keeps the other awake. It is also common for people to get defensive when told they snore; some even deny it, never suspecting they have a deeper underlying problem.

When Should You Seek Help?

So how do you know when it is time to investigate? Start by reflecting (or asking your bed partner) whether you snore loudly and often. Has anyone noticed pauses in your breathing at night? Do you wake up with a headache or dry mouth? Do you feel foggy or doze off during the day, especially while reading or watching TV? If the answer to any of these is yes, it is worth seeing a doctor. A home sleep study or a more detailed in-clinic test can confirm whether sleep apnoea is to blame.

Fortunately, there are ways to address this. If diagnosed, treatment options can include lifestyle changes such as losing weight, reducing or stopping alcohol consumption, and adjusting your sleeping position. More advanced solutions may involve using a CPAP (continuous positive airway pressure) machine, which helps keep your airway open, or dental devices fitted by a specialist. The most important thing is not to ignore the signs and assume you are just a bad sleeper.

Putting It into Practice

- If you or your partner notice loud or frequent snoring, take it seriously; it could be more than just noise.
- Keep a sleep journal or use a snore-tracking app for a few nights. Record how you feel during the day.
- If sleep apnoea is suspected, a sleep study (polysomnography) is the gold standard. There are also home-based options available.
- Depending on the severity, treatment might involve lifestyle changes, a CPAP machine (for moderate to severe cases), or dental devices that keep your airway open.
- Reducing alcohol, losing excess weight, and sleeping on your side instead of your back can all help reduce snoring.

You've Got This

Do not ignore snoring or let embarrassment prevent you from seeking help. You deserve restful sleep and the chance to wake up feeling truly refreshed. Whether it involves a minor lifestyle change or professional evaluation, taking action today can improve your quality of life.

5

Sleep and Mental Health: A Two-Way Street

When I first talked to Sneha, a high-achieving executive in her late 30s, she described her mind as 'a browser with 37 tabs open simultaneously'. She had been struggling with insomnia for years. 'I cannot remember the last time I slept through the night without waking up in a panic about some deadline,' she admitted. What struck me was not just her sleep deprivation, but how she described her emotional state: constant worry, irritability, trouble focusing, and an overwhelming feeling that her mind was working against her.

What Sneha was experiencing illustrates one of the most overlooked links between sleep and mental well-being. Poor sleep worsens anxiety and depression, which then further disrupts sleep, creating a cycle that can feel impossible to break.

The Neurological Dance

Sleep deprivation affects the amygdala, the brain's emotional processing centre. Neuroimaging studies show that even one night of insufficient sleep can increase amygdala reactivity by up to 60 per cent, making you much more responsive to negative stimuli. Meanwhile, the prefrontal cortex (the front of the brain), responsible for rational thinking and emotional regulation, becomes less active when you are sleep deprived.

This neurobiological shift creates the perfect storm: heightened emotional reactivity combined with a reduced ability to regulate those emotions. It is like driving a car with an overly sensitive accelerator and worn-out brakes.

The relationship also works in reverse. Anxiety and depression can disrupt the natural progression through sleep stages. People with anxiety typically experience less slow-wave sleep (your deepest, most restorative sleep phase) and more fragmented REM sleep. Those with depression may enter REM sleep too early and stay in that state for too long. This worsens negative thought patterns and emotional instability.

The Stress Hormone Connection

Cortisol, your main stress hormone, is essential in this process. Normally, cortisol follows a clear 24-hour rhythm: it peaks in the morning to help you wake up, gradually declines throughout the day, and reaches its lowest point at night to allow sleep.

Chronic stress and anxiety interfere with this pattern. Many people with anxiety have elevated cortisol levels that remain high into the evening, making it physiologically difficult to fall asleep. This imbalance not only affects how quickly you fall asleep but also causes fragmented sleep, leading to waking up in the middle of the night and experiencing early-morning insomnia more often.

Similarly, depression is often marked by a flattened cortisol rhythm. It does not rise appropriately in the morning or fall sufficiently at night. This hormonal flatline contributes to both the sleep problems and the daytime fatigue commonly seen in depression.

Breaking the Cycle

Understanding the relationship between sleep and mental health is the first step towards reclaiming both. Improvement in one often leads to progress in the other. Aim for a strategy that gently tackles both.

Create a consistent sleep schedule and follow it even on the weekends. A simple wind-down ritual can help relax your nervous system before bed. Keep your bedroom cool, quiet, and dark to support rest. Dimming blue light at least 90 minutes before sleep helps reset your circadian clock.

Think of mental health practices like sleep medicine. Try worry journalling not at bedtime but before dinner to give anxious thoughts a place to rest. Diaphragmatic (belly) breathing, practised during the day, activates the parasympathetic (calming) nervous system. Challenge and change any thoughts that scare you. Many are surprised by how quickly a small positive change – such as less bedtime scrolling, deeper breaths, or improved light hygiene – can create a ripple throughout the system.

When to Seek Professional Help

Lifestyle strategies are powerful but not a substitute for professional intervention when necessary. Contact a professional if your sleep issues persist despite consistent efforts, or if you experience intense sleep-onset anxiety, panic attacks, or persistent morning dread. If alcohol or substances have become your nightly crutch, or if your insomnia is related to trauma or major life changes, seeking professional help can guide you to a safer and more effective reset.

The Microbiome Connection

And just when you thought the sleep–mental health relationship could not get more interesting, here comes your gut. The gut–brain axis, the biochemical conversation between your digestive system and nervous system, plays a crucial role in how your mood and sleep tend to be.

Your gut microbiome helps regulate neurotransmitters like serotonin and GABA, directly affecting both mood and sleep quality. Supporting gut health through fermented foods, a variety of plant-based foods, and stress reduction can improve both sleep quality and emotional resilience. It is another way to gently influence this cycle from within.

You've Got This

Understanding sleep and mental health as two sides of the same coin liberates you from the trap of fixing one while ignoring the other. Whether your starting point is sleep disruption or emotional distress, recognising the bidirectional relationship opens multiple pathways for intervention. The cycle can become virtuous instead of vicious, with better sleep leading to improved emotional regulation, which enables even better sleep, creating an upward spiral of well-being.

Part VII

Mind Matters

1. The Mind–Body Health Link You Cannot Ignore
2. Managing Stress: Your Toolkit for Calm in a Chaotic World
3. The Dopamine Dance: Pleasure, Motivation, and Well-Being
4. Breaking Free from Social Anxiety
5. Health Anxiety: When Body Awareness Becomes Fear
6. The Science of Self-Reflection
7. The Science of Habit Formation: How to Build Healthy Habits That Stick
8. Digital Detox, Because Offline Is the New Luxury
9. Running on Empty: How to Recognise and Recover from Burnout
10. Laughter, Ritual, Belonging: The Science of Social Wellness

1

The Mind–Body Health Link You Cannot Ignore

The way your stomach tightens before a difficult conversation, or your heart races when anxiety takes hold, or you feel like you are physically sick when you fight with a loved one – these are not just manifestations of stress. These are signs that your mental and physical health are constantly communicating, whether you are paying attention or not.

Yet, in modern life, we often behave as if the brain and body live in separate spaces. We go to the gym for our bodies and use meditation apps for our minds. But in reality, they are roommates, constantly interacting and influencing one another, for better or worse.

Let us examine what science reveals about this powerful mind–body connection, and what you can do with that knowledge.

The Science Behind the Mind–Body Connection

When we experience stress, the hypothalamic-pituitary-adrenal (HPA) axis gets activated, releasing the stress hormone cortisol. Cortisol, in small doses, is essential for regulating blood sugar, metabolism, and our immune response. It provides the necessary energy and alertness needed for daily functioning, acting as a natural alarm system. However, chronic stress results in chronically elevated cortisol, which is harmful. It causes the heart rate and blood pressure to stay elevated, weakens the immune system, and disrupts sleep. Studies consistently show that people with chronic stress are at higher risk for cardiovascular disease.[1]

Depression, too, has ripple effects beyond just mood. It can sap your drive to move, eat well, or take care of yourself. A major 2017 study in *The Lancet* found that people with depression have a

37 per cent higher risk of developing type 2 diabetes.[2] Anxiety may keep you wired at night and exhausted during the day, wearing down your body over time. It can also increase inflammation, a major player in autoimmune disorders and other chronic illnesses.

This is both psychological and physiological. Mental states can alter hormonal signals, immune responses, and even how your gut functions.

The Gut–Brain Axis: A Two-Way Street

One of the most fascinating areas of research today is the link between your brain and gut, a relationship often described as a 'second brain' scenario. Your gut roughly contains 100 trillion microbes that affect not only digestion but also mood, immunity, and inflammation. Stress and poor mental health can reduce microbial diversity, leading to gut dysbiosis. This imbalance contributes to inflammation and worsens both mental and physical health. The vagus nerve, a major communication channel between the gut and brain, plays a critical role here. When this pathway is disrupted, symptoms can appear anywhere – mood swings, digestive issues, fatigue, even skin flare-ups.

The Silver Lining

We can take comfort in the fact that positive mental health can work wonders for your body. Studies show that optimism and mindfulness go beyond just lifting your spirits. They lower blood pressure and reduce the risk of heart disease.[3] Happiness and strong social connections can even accelerate recovery after surgery, thanks to decreased stress and inflammation. When you feel good mentally, your body produces beneficial chemicals like serotonin, which eases pain and boosts immunity. It is like giving your health a natural upgrade.

What You Can Do About It

Ready to put this into action? We will walk through some simple steps:
- Start with mindfulness. Five minutes of deep breathing daily (with exhalations longer than inhalations) can reduce cortisol and stress.

- Move more. Exercise offers a double benefit by lifting your mood and strengthening your body. Aim for 30 minutes of exercise each day. Play a game you enjoy, dance to a YouTube video, play with your pet, or just take a walk.
- Connect socially. Call a friend, cuddle your dog, or spend time with loved ones. Social bonds act as a shield against stress.
- Guard your sleep routine. Recharge both mind and body. If you are struggling, seek support through therapy or consult a sleep specialist.

Small moves like these add up, linking mental peace to physical well-being.

Your mind and body are a team. Stress, depression, or anxiety can throw them out of sync, increasing the risk of heart problems, diabetes, and more. When you nurture your mental health, your body reaps the rewards – lower disease risk, faster recovery, and more energy to live your life.

Putting It into Practice

Here are two practical ways to start today:
- Spend 5 to 10 minutes each day practising mindfulness. This could involve deep breathing, a short meditation, or a quiet walk (without your phone) where you tune into your senses.
- If you are feeling overwhelmed by stress, talk to a trusted friend, or consider speaking with a mental health professional.

Recommended reading

- *The Body Keeps the Score: Mind, Brain and Body in the Transformation of Trauma* by Bessel van der Kolk

You've Got This

Mental and physical health are not two separate goals. They are intertwined systems, each shaping the other in real time. When you nurture your mind, your body becomes stronger, more resilient, and better equipped to handle life's challenges.

Begin with where you are, using what you can handle. Every step you take to nurture your mental well-being will also improve your physical health.

2

Managing Stress: Your Toolkit for Calm in a Chaotic World

If I had to distil the blueprint of good health into just four foundational pillars, stress management would undoubtedly be one of them, right alongside food, movement, and sleep.

Yet, unlike trending diets or fitness routines, stress rarely receives the attention it deserves. Most of us treat chronic stress like background noise – always present, rarely acknowledged, and somehow normalised. While a short burst of stress can be helpful, even life-saving, living in a state of constant overwhelm is not a badge of honour. It quietly erodes our health by disrupting sleep, fuelling inflammation, and impairing cognitive function.

But we have good news. Stress management is not some elusive, elite-level skill. It is completely doable, with the right tools and consistent practice.

Understanding the Stress Response

Stress is the body's natural reaction to a perceived threat. When faced with a challenge, your brain triggers a chain reaction: adrenaline spikes, cortisol levels rise, and your body prepares for fight or flight. In short bursts, this response is protective. However, if it remains day after day, month after month, it can disrupt your health.

At the core of this stress response is the HPA axis (hypothalamic-pituitary-adrenal axis), which is your body's built-in alarm system responsible for this cascade.

- **Step 1**: The hypothalamus releases CRH (corticotropin-releasing hormone).
- **Step 2**: This stimulates the pituitary gland to release ACTH (adrenocorticotropic hormone).

- **Step 3**: ACTH signals the adrenal glands to release cortisol, the main stress hormone.

Cortisol is not inherently bad. But when this system remains activated for too long, it becomes imbalanced. And that is when problems start.

Six Practical Tools for Managing Stress

Breathing

Your breath is your built-in stress regulator and is always available to you, no matter where you are. Slow, deep breathing activates the parasympathetic nervous system (your rest-and-digest mode), helping to counteract the effects of chronic cortisol.

Some effective techniques include the following:
- **Diaphragmatic breathing**: Place one hand on your chest and the other on your abdomen. Breathe so that only your abdomen rises and falls. This calms the nervous system and slows the heart rate.
- **4-7-8 breathing**: Inhale for 4 counts, hold for 7, exhale for 8. This technique is especially helpful before bedtime.
- **Box breathing**: Inhale–hold–exhale–hold, each for 4 counts. Used by athletes and high performers to stay centred under pressure.
- **Cyclic sighing**: This is a technique shown in recent research to lower the respiratory rate and improve mood by doing longer exhalations.

Meditation

Meditation helps calm the mind and cultivate awareness of the present moment. It reduces stress, improves emotional regulation, and supports mental clarity.

Explore different styles (many of which are available for free on YouTube) and see what resonates with you.
- **Mindfulness meditation**: Paying attention to your thoughts without judgement. Ideal for beginners and effective for managing anxiety.

- **Loving-kindness meditation**: Cultivating compassion for yourself and others, especially powerful for those who struggle with self-criticism.
- **Transcendental meditation**: Uses a mantra to calm the mind and access a deeper state of rest.
- **Guided meditation**: Practising guided meditation through apps like Calm and Headspace or through YouTube videos is a great way for beginners to get started.

Combine three to five minutes of breathwork with meditation for a synergistic effect.

Physical activity

Exercise is one of the most effective stress regulators. It helps metabolise excess cortisol and releases feel-good chemicals like serotonin and endorphins.
- Moderate-intensity activities (like walking, swimming, and cycling) soothe the nervous system.
- Strength training enhances both physical and mental resilience.
- Movement-based mindfulness (like yoga, Tai Chi, or Qigong) combines the best of physical activity and meditation.

Social connection

Loneliness and isolation exacerbate stress. Strong social connections serve as a shield against stress. Spending time with loved ones or pets boosts oxytocin, which counteracts cortisol. Support groups, therapy, or even casual social interactions can help reduce stress levels.

Sleep optimisation

Chronic stress interferes with sleep, and poor sleep increases stress, creating a vicious cycle. Establishing a bedtime routine (such as no screens, dim lighting, and relaxation techniques) helps regulate cortisol. Managing sleep hygiene (consistent sleep–wake times, avoiding stimulants before bed) improves stress resilience.

Journalling

Putting your thoughts on paper can be therapeutic. Whether you are writing out your worries or listing things you are grateful for,

journalling can help you manage stress and see challenges in a new light.
- **Worry dump**: Write out what is on your mind, not for solutions, just to vent.
- **Gratitude journalling**: Listing three good things each day can help your brain shift away from a problem-focused mindset.
- **Applying principles of cognitive behavioural therapy (CBT)**: Learn to identify and challenge distorted thinking patterns. (A therapist or even an online course can help with this.)

Putting It into Practice

- Start small. Begin meditation and breathwork with short sessions, and gradually increase the duration as your comfort improves.
- Start a gratitude and brain-dump journal.
- Stay consistent with your sleep routine.

You've Got This

You do not need to overhaul your life to feel better. Start small – take a deep breath or go for a short walk – and tackle stress a few mindful moments at a time.

3

The Dopamine Dance: Pleasure, Motivation, and Well-Being

A new, highly anticipated series had just dropped on Netflix. At 10 p.m., Amit told himself he would watch just one episode before bed. But as the credits rolled, the next one auto-played, and the cliffhanger was too good to ignore. 'Just one more,' he told himself. By the time he looked up, it was 2 a.m.

What kept him hooked was more than the plot line. It was dopamine, the brain's anticipation-and-reward chemical, which was pulling the strings.

Dopamine plays a crucial role in motivation, reward, and pleasure. However, this neurotransmitter is essential for various bodily functions, impacting our health and well-being in multifaceted ways.

Often dubbed the 'feel-good' neurotransmitter, dopamine's influence extends far beyond simple gratification. It shapes motivation, habit formation, focus, and movement. Its ripple effects reach deep into our everyday choices and health.

Understanding Dopamine

Dopamine is a chemical messenger produced in several regions of the brain, including the substantia nigra and the ventral tegmental area (VTA). It transmits signals between nerve cells and is integral to several vital physiological processes, including the following:

- **Mood regulation**: Dopamine helps produce feelings of pleasure and satisfaction. Imbalances are often associated with mood disorders such as depression.
- **Movement control**: It plays a key role in coordinating movement. In Parkinson's disease, the loss of dopamine-

producing neurons in the substantia nigra causes tremors, rigidity, and difficulties with movement.
- **Cognitive functions**: Dopamine influences learning, attention, and decision-making. Balanced levels are essential for focus, mental flexibility, and working memory.

The Dopamine Effect: Why the Same Reward Feels Less Exciting Over Time

Ever noticed how the first bite of your favourite dessert is pure bliss, but the next few are just … okay? Or how the excitement of a new phone fades in a few days, leaving you looking for the next upgrade? That is dopamine working behind the scenes, not just in giving you pleasure, but in pushing you towards new rewards.

A fascinating study published in 2025 found that dopamine actively reduces the value of past rewards in our memory.[4] In simple terms, once we experience something pleasurable, our brain begins to downplay its significance over time, encouraging us to seek out new experiences.

This mechanism explains the following common situations in everyday life: the first victory in a game feels exhilarating, but after repeated wins, it loses its thrill. Shopping for something new is exciting, but even by the time you receive the parcel, the excitement has faded.

People often pursue new relationships, experiences, or achievements instead of being content with what they already have. This dopamine-driven urge helped our ancestors survive and adapt by promoting exploration, innovation, and risk-taking. But in the modern world, it can manifest as impulse buying, addiction, and hours lost to mindless scrolling.

The good news is that understanding how dopamine works helps us manage it more effectively, choosing long-term fulfilment over fleeting highs.

Dopamine Imbalances

Too little or too much dopamine can throw the brain off balance.
- **Dopamine deficiency**: When dopamine levels drop too low, you might feel apathetic, unmotivated, fatigued, or even depressed. It is also connected to movement disorders like

Parkinson's disease and can impair memory and focus over time.
- **Dopamine excess**: Conversely, an overload of dopamine, often caused by addictive substances, compulsive behaviours, or overstimulation, can result in impulsive decisions, risky behaviours, and addictive patterns that are difficult to break.

How to Keep Dopamine in Balance

Thankfully, several everyday habits can help keep dopamine levels within a healthy range:
- **Exercise**: Physical activity triggers dopamine release and is associated with better mood and sharper thinking.
- **Nutrition**: Foods rich in tyrosine, an amino acid that helps produce dopamine, can support healthy levels. For example: almonds, bananas, avocados, eggs, and tofu.
- **Sleep**: Dopamine receptors need rest too. Poor or insufficient sleep disrupts dopamine signalling, often leading to brain fog, irritability, or low motivation.
- **Mindfulness and meditation**: These soothe the nervous system and may help recalibrate dopamine pathways by reducing chronic stress.
- **Cold exposure**: Cold showers and exposure to cold temperatures can increase dopamine levels.
- **Sunlight**: Natural light, especially in the morning, supports dopamine production and helps regulate your circadian rhythm.

Putting It into Practice

- Put your phone down and take a 15-minute walk. Bonus points if it is outdoors. Moving around and sunlight create a dopamine-friendly combo.
- Enjoy a handful of almonds or a banana. Easy fuel for your brain's chemicals.
- Meet a friend for a quick chat or coffee. Meaningful connection also triggers dopamine.

Recommended reading
- *Dopamine Detox: A Short Guide to Remove Distractions and Get Your Brain to Do Hard Things* by Thibaut Meurisse

- *Dopamine Nation: Finding Balance in the Age of Indulgence* by Dr Anna Lembke

You've Got This

Understanding dopamine helps you work in tune with your brain. When you support dopamine through healthy, balanced habits, you are more likely to feel focused, calm, and content, instead of constantly chasing the next hit of excitement.

4

Breaking Free from Social Anxiety

Rohan received an invitation to his cousin's wedding. His initial reaction was not excitement but panic. The thought of making small talk with distant relatives, being introduced to strangers, and figuring out what to do in a crowded room made his stomach turn. He spent days crafting excuses to avoid going, even though a part of him wanted to be there.

This is an example of social anxiety disorder (SAD), an intense fear of social situations that leads to avoidance and distress. Social anxiety is much more than just shyness. It is a persistent, often paralysing fear of being judged, criticised, or humiliated. This fear can significantly affect personal relationships, career advancement, and overall well-being.

In everyday conversation, 'social anxiety' is often used loosely to mean feeling awkward or uneasy around others. But the actual clinical condition is rooted in psychology and biology and is far more serious.

Understanding Social Anxiety

SAD involves a persistent fear of being judged, embarrassed, or humiliated in social settings. This fear can manifest in physical symptoms such as sweating, trembling, rapid heartbeat, and even nausea. Why does it happen?

Several factors can contribute to the development of social anxiety:
- **Cognitive factors**: Negative thought patterns like 'everyone is judging me' or 'I am not likeable' fuel avoidance behaviours, which in turn reinforce the anxiety.
- **Biological factors**: Genetics and neurochemical imbalances can make some people more prone to developing SAD.

- **Environmental factors**: Experiences like bullying, rejection, or prolonged isolation (such as during the COVID-19 pandemic) can heighten vulnerability.

Evidence-Based Strategies to Overcome Social Anxiety

Managing social anxiety requires a multifaceted approach that targets both the mind and behaviour. With the right tools, support, and consistent practice, it is possible to break the cycle of fear and feel confident in social situations.

If social anxiety significantly affects your work or relationships, seeking professional help is essential.

- **Cognitive behavioural therapy**: CBT is one of the most effective treatments for SAD. It helps individuals identify and challenge irrational thoughts while developing healthier coping mechanisms.
- **Exposure therapy**: A subset of CBT, this method involves gradually and repeatedly exposing individuals to feared social situations to help build their resilience. Innovations like virtual reality therapy now allow people to practise in safe, controlled environments.
- **Social skills training**: Learning practical skills like initiating conversations and maintaining eye contact can significantly improve social interactions.
- **Mindfulness-based interventions**: Techniques such as meditation and deep breathing can help lower overall anxiety and increase presence and awareness.
- **Medications**: In some cases, medications such as selective serotonin reuptake inhibitors (SSRIs) or serotonin-norepinephrine reuptake inhibitors (SNRIs) may be prescribed when therapy alone is not enough.

Lifestyle Modifications

Lifestyle changes can complement therapy or serve as an initial step for mild to moderate cases:
- **Exercise regularly**: Physical activity lowers stress hormones and boosts mood.
- **Get enough sleep**: Rest is crucial for emotional regulation and cognitive clarity.

- **Join a support group**: Sharing experiences with others facing similar challenges can be validating and helpful.

Putting It into Practice

- **Start small**: Ease into low-pressure social situations and work your way up.
- **Be kind to yourself**: Remind yourself that social anxiety is common and that most people are focused on themselves, not on judging you.
- **Try grounding exercises**: Use techniques like the 5-4-3-2-1 method (5 things you can see, 4 things you can touch, 3 things you hear, 2 things you smell, 1 thing you taste) to anchor yourself in the moment when anxiety spikes.

Recommended reading

- *How to Be Yourself: Quiet Your Inner Critic and Rise Above Social Anxiety* by Ellen Hendriksen
- *The Solution to Social Anxiety: Break Free from the Shyness That Holds You Back* by Dr Aziz Gazipura

You've Got This

Social anxiety can feel overwhelming, but it does not have to control your life. With time, the right tools, and self-compassion, it becomes manageable. You are not alone, and every small step forward matters. Learning to feel more at ease in social settings is a journey, and patience with yourself is just as important as any technique.

5

Health Anxiety: When Body Awareness Becomes Fear

Neha, a 35-year-old working mother, began experiencing dull headaches once or twice a week. At first, she attributed them to stress. But as the weeks went by, worry set in – what if it was something more serious? A late-night internet search led her to articles about brain tumours, and panic took hold. She began tracking every detail of her headaches: timing, duration, intensity, and frequency. She avoided bright lights, felt dizzy at times, and each recurrence of pain amplified her anxiety. Even after a normal MRI, she could not shake her fear. What if something had been missed?

Ravi, a 40-year-old marathon runner, was cooling down after a run when he felt a strange flutter in his chest. It was not the first time, but this time it triggered a wave of worry. He checked his pulse and ECG on his smartwatch, which gave him a clean chit. But his worry did not subside, and he went straight for a cardiologist's evaluation. Even though all his tests came back normal, over the next few months Ravi became hyper-aware of his heartbeat, checking his heart rate multiple times a day, and the stress started affecting the quality of his life.

That flutter in your chest, the persistent headache, the unfamiliar stomach sensation – for most people, these are everyday annoyances. But for someone with health anxiety, even normal bodily signals can spiral into overwhelming fear, trapping them in a cycle that is hard to break.

What Is Health Anxiety?

Health anxiety, once called hypochondriasis, occurs when your body's normal sensations become exaggerated. A flutter in your chest, headache or dizziness, or even digestive issues all become potential signs of something catastrophic. Between 2 and 13 per cent of people experience this condition. Among those who frequently visit clinics and hospitals, that percentage increases to 7–19.9 per cent.[5]

Think of it as your body's alarm system stuck on high alert, like a car alarm that goes off even when someone is 10 m away.

How It Shows Up in Everyday Life

Let me share a personal experience. I naturally have a higher resting heart rate, and, for a while, that alone made me anxious. I found myself obsessively checking my heart rate on my Apple Watch, sometimes even checking the ECG when I felt some discomfort. Everything was normal, and yet my mind kept asking, 'Could something be wrong?'

After COVID-19, these thoughts became louder. Heart attacks in young people made the news, and every little thud in my chest felt like a potential obituary. In six months, I saw my cardiologist three times. Each visit ended with the same calm reassurance: 'You are fine.' Eventually, I even underwent a CT angiography, not because it was medically necessary, but because a trusted cardiologist friend suggested it might help my mind catch up with my body.

I am sharing this because I want you to know you are not alone. Health anxiety is more common than we realise.

The Four Faces of Health Anxiety

Health anxiety manifests in the following four aspects of our lives.

In our thoughts:

- A simple headache feels like a brain tumour
- A post-workout heart rate spike causes panic about heart disease
- A regular viral fever feels like dengue or worse

In our behaviours:

- Compulsive symptom checking, like pulse, temperature, and lumps
- Seeking constant reassurance from doctors, friends, and the internet

- Avoiding triggers like hospitals or health news
- Getting 'just in case' medical tests done
- Falling into the Google black hole

In our bodies:

- A heightened awareness of normal bodily sensations
- Physical symptoms of anxiety (racing heart, muscle tension) are mistaken for disease
- Chronic tension that ironically creates more symptoms

In our relationships:

- Frequently seeking reassurance from loved ones
- Missing out on activities due to health worries
- Straining relationships with repeated health concerns

The Digital Age and Health Anxiety

We used to consult doctors. Now we consult Google (or ChatGPT). The result is a new condition: cyberchondria, the infinite scroll of symptom checking, aggravated by articles that start with '10 signs you might have…' and end with 'see your doctor immediately'.

The modern health-tech dream of wearables, trackers, and apps promised us control. However, what it often delivers is hypervigilance. Smartwatches, step counters, and sleep analysers help some people, but for others, they generate a constant state of bodily surveillance that borders on obsession.

And then there is the healthcare system, which, with its tests-on-demand culture and no-time-for-conversation appointments, sometimes reinforces our worst fears. If you have ever felt rushed, dismissed, or over-tested, you know what I mean.

Breaking the Cycle

There are many approaches you can take to break out of the cycle of health anxiety. CBT, mindfulness practices, and making small changes in your daily life can help you in many ways.

CBT is the gold standard. It helps you:
- Identify catastrophic thinking and question it
- Gently expose yourself to feared sensations (like feeling your heart race during exercise and learning that it is okay)

- Run mini 'experiments' to test if your anxious predictions really come true

Mindfulness approaches help you:
- Observe bodily sensations without judgement
- Accept uncertainty about health (a challenging but crucial skill) – knowing that health is not an all-or-nothing phenomenon and variations happen all the time
- Practise present-moment awareness rather than worrying about the future

Daily anchors that help:
- Limit body checking and online symptom research
- Use only reliable sources, and only at specific times
- Fill your day with engaging, outward-focused activities like music, gardening, painting, or long walks
- Take care of your body through exercise, sleep, and real food, not through over-monitoring

Putting It into Practice

If health anxiety is taking over your day, it is time to get help. Therapy can make a big difference. Do not wait until it is bad enough. Even mild health anxiety deserves attention.

For me, the biggest change happened when I decided to stop wearing my smartwatch altogether, so I could lead my days without hyper self-monitoring.

You've Got This

Sometimes, the issue is not your body but the culture of fear, hyper-vigilance, and overdiagnosis that we are all immersed in. Understanding this and taking a step back may be the healthiest choice of all.

6

The Science of Self-Reflection

Can journalling help you achieve better health?

When was the last time you wrote something with a pen? Not a signature, not a to-do list, but actual thoughts written down using pen and paper. In a world that encourages us to be fast, reactive, and screen-bound, journalling with actual pen and paper feels almost rebellious. It is a daily chance to slow down, reflect, and simply be human.

My interest in journalling began at the end of 2023, not driven by any big self-improvement goal but by a desire to feel more centred. I thought it might help add structure to a chaotic work–life balance, ease my tendency to overthink, and promote a slower, more mindful way of living. What I discovered was that journalling, especially when done by hand, is not just a tool to stay organised; it is a deeply therapeutic ritual that strengthens mental health, supports physical well-being, and offers a private, judgement-free space to process life as it unfolds.

Different Ways to Journal

If the only things you have ever written down are grocery lists or reminders, you will be in for a surprise. Journalling comes in many forms, and there is no one-size-fits-all approach. Here are a few common types, each serving a different purpose:

Morning Pages

Introduced by Julia Cameron in *The Artist's Way*, Morning Pages involve writing three pages of stream-of-consciousness every morning. This unfiltered brain dump helps clear mental clutter, spark creativity, and create space for self-awareness. There is no structure, no audience, just you and your thoughts.

Gratitude journal

Far from the cliched 'I am grateful for family, food, and friends', a meaningful gratitude practice encourages you to look deeper. What made you smile today? What did you almost miss but are glad you noticed? This journal helps train your brain to recognise the good, even on tough days, gradually transforming your outlook over time.

Art journal

Combining visuals and words, an art journal is for those moments when language does not quite suffice. Whether you are sketching a cafe scene, pasting in a museum ticket, or doodling your feelings, it is a place to document life creatively, being fully present in the moment.

Food journal

Not every food journal needs to focus on counting calories. Try documenting how you ate instead of just what. Where were you? What was your mood? How did you feel after the meal? Over time, these patterns offer clues to your relationship with food and help you make more mindful choices.

Bullet journal

The bullet journal system – a planner, diary, and to-do list all combined – developed by Ryder Carroll, is ideal for those who crave structure with flexibility. Using short-form notes, symbols, and modular sections, it can hold everything from habit trackers to personal reflections.

What Journalling Does for Your Health

It may seem unlikely that a simple notebook could have measurable health effects, but research suggests otherwise. Journalling influences both mental and physical health in surprising ways:

- Reduces stress by offering an emotional outlet[6]
- Improves mood through increased mindfulness and emotional clarity[7]
- Strengthens immunity by reducing stress-related inflammation
- Improves sleep – expressive writing before bed has been shown to ease cognitive overload[8]

- Supports healing – even physical wounds seem to heal faster in people who journal regularly
- Clarity of goals and priorities – writing down your goals and reviewing them regularly boosts your chances of achieving them[9]

Neuroscientist Andrew Huberman, in his podcast episode 'A Science-Supported Journalling Protocol to Improve Mental and Physical Health', highlights journalling's impact on everything from chronic pain and fibromyalgia to anxiety and insomnia. In one study he references, participants wrote about traumatic or emotional experiences for just 15 to 20 minutes daily over several days and experienced notable health benefits.

How to Journal

- **Just get started**: If you have never journaled before, it may seem intimidating. The key is to begin without worrying about grammar, handwriting, or language. Your journal is only for you. If your mind feels blank initially, sit down and write anyway. Over time, your thoughts will flow more freely.
- **Be consistent**: Some people prefer to journal in the morning, others before bed, and some carry a pocket notebook throughout the day. If you are new, start with 'one line a day'. This simple habit builds consistency and makes journalling feel effortless over time.
- **Make it enjoyable**: Create a journalling ritual you look forward to. Choose a quiet space, light a candle, or play calming music. While you do not need fancy stationery, using a notebook and pen you love can make the practice more inviting.
- **Combine words and visuals**: Your journal can include sketches, doodles, pasted ticket stubs, cafe receipts, or stickers. Including visual elements can make the experience more engaging and personal.
- **Focus on feelings and reflections**: Instead of merely documenting events, explore how they made you feel. Reflecting on emotions fosters deeper self-awareness and personal growth.

Putting It into Practice

- Keep a notebook and pen handy near your bed or wherever else you feel comfortable writing from.
- Write a few lines every day that include three things you were grateful for during the day and a couple of reflections from the day.

Recommended reading

- *The Artist's Way* by Julia Cameron

You've Got This

Journalling will not fix everything, but it offers something rare in today's world – a pause and relief from doomscrolling. It is a chance to check in with yourself, free and unfiltered. Over time, that pause becomes a mirror, a compass, and a powerful path to healing. So, if you are seeking a tool to improve your health – not just mental or physical, but something more integrated – consider this your invitation to start writing.

7

The Science of Habit Formation: How to Build Healthy Habits That Stick

Most of us have tried the 'new year, new me' routine, aiming to finally master meditation or commit to the gym. We have been there, full of hope, only to see our resolutions crumble like stale cake in just days or weeks.

Take Sarita, for example, who struggled with chronic fatigue and tried countless remedies to no avail. But things only started to change when she began building small, manageable habits: a 10-minute morning walk, a nutrient-dense breakfast, and a consistent bedtime. Her energy levels began to improve.

So why do we need habits? And why, as fully grown adults, are we still struggling with forming habits? Shouldn't we have figured this out by now?

The truth is, our adult brains are highly adaptable. Neuroplasticity, which is the brain's ability to form new neural connections, remains active throughout our lives. However, we also battle against decades of ingrained patterns: some helpful, others harmful. Our existing routines, associations, and neural pathways do not always make room for change.

And then there is the modern world. We live in an attention economy. Distractions are everywhere – social media, work pressures, and easy access to hyper-palatable food all steal our attention and impulses. These forces often work against the very changes we are trying to make.

That is why building healthy habits is a form of resistance – a way to take back control in a world set on controlling your behaviour. It is about making your daily actions match your long-term goals and well-being.

Understanding the Habit Loop

At the heart of habit formation is what Charles Duhigg describes in *The Power of Habit* as the habit loop, a neurological cycle that controls all our routines:
- **Cue (Trigger)**: The signal that initiates the behaviour. This can be a specific time of the day, location, emotional state, or event.
- **Routine (Behaviour)**: The habit itself – what you do in response to the cue.
- **Reward (Reinforcement)**: The positive outcome your brain receives, which strengthens the loop.

Here is a relatable example:
- **Cue**: Opening Netflix after a long day and craving some relaxation.
- **Routine**: Reaching for a bag of chips.
- **Reward**: The comforting crunch and the dopamine boost from the show and the food.

Your brain quickly associates the cue (Netflix) with the routine (snacking), and because the reward feels good, it automates the behaviour.

This same loop governs *both* unhealthy and healthy habits. However, developing positive habits presents its own distinct challenges.

Why Healthy Habits Are Harder

- **Delayed gratification**: Healthy habits usually provide long-term benefits rather than instant payoffs. That quinoa salad will not give you a dopamine spike like a samosa.
- **Discomfort**: Exercising, sleeping early, or eating mindfully can initially feel boring, exhausting, or demanding too much effort – things your brain naturally wants to avoid.
- **Social and environmental triggers**: Junk food is everywhere. Friends may encourage 'just one drink'. Your environment often reinforces old habits, not new ones.
- **Competing neural pathways**: You are not only forming a new habit but also working against an older, stronger one that has been deeply embedded over the years.

How to Build Habits That Last

Here is a step-by-step plan that aligns with how your brain actually works:

- **Be specific**: Replace vague goals like 'get fitter' with 'walk for 30 minutes every morning'.
- **Choose a cue**: Attach it to something you already do, like 'after brushing my teeth' or 'once I drop my kid at the bus stop'.
- **Start small**: Make the action ridiculously easy. Two minutes of meditation. Two push-ups. One glass of water.
- **Choose your reward**: A gold star on a tracker, a small treat, or 15 minutes of watching your favourite YouTube channel. Make the brain want to repeat it.
- **Use If-Then planning**: For example, 'If it is 7 a.m., I go for a walk', 'If I turn on Netflix, I will brew a cup of herbal tea instead of opening a bag of chips'. This reinforces the cue–routine link.
- **Track it**: Use a habit tracker, app, or journal. Seeing your consistent efforts visually can be incredibly motivating.
- **Iterate weekly**: If something does not work, tweak it. Change the time, the trigger, the reward, but do not abandon the process.
- **Celebrate small wins**: Each successful repetition reinforces the loop. Acknowledge it. That is how motivation builds.

Putting It into Practice

Like my friend Ashdin Doctor, a habit coach, says:
- Pick the ridiculously smallest thing.
- Make it very easy to do.
- Do not skip two days in a row.

Recommended reading

- *Atomic Habits: An Easy and Proven Way to Build Good Habits and Break Bad Ones* by James Clear
- *Change Your Habits, Change Your Life: Your Guide to an Awesome Life* by Ashdin Doctor

You've Got This

Every lasting change begins with one small, consistent action. Be patient with yourself.

Habits take time, but each repetition is proof that you're getting closer to your goal.

8

Digital Detox, Because Offline Is the New Luxury

When I first heard the term *nomophobia* over a decade ago, I laughed. Who could possibly be afraid of being without their mobile phone or losing mobile connection?

Coined during a 2008 UK Post Office study evaluating mobile phone users' anxieties, the portmanteau of *no-mobile-phone-phobia* seemed an amusing exaggeration at the time. But as smartphones gradually integrated into the fabric of our daily lives – serving as our cameras, calendars, alarm clocks, entertainment centres, and even our mirrors – nomophobia has evolved into something very real. Today, it is not so much a phobia as it is a near-universal condition.

As screen time soars for individuals globally, the real question is not how much we are glued to our devices but what we are sacrificing in exchange and what it will take to regain our time, attention, and well-being.

The Global Screen Time Epidemic

By 2023, adult screen time worldwide surpassed seven hours per day, with countries like the US and the Philippines averaging more than nine hours daily. What was already a concerning trend accelerated sharply during the pandemic. Lockdowns, isolation, and the shift to remote work and online schooling blurred the lines between work, rest, and leisure.

This shift represents more than a change in behaviour. It is a cultural transformation where digital interaction increasingly replaces face-to-face connection and real-world engagement.

What Are We Missing Out On?

When six to nine hours of our waking life are spent in front of screens, it is clear that we are missing out on something.

While technology offers undeniable benefits like convenience, global connectivity, and instant information, it also reduces time spent outdoors, engaging in physical activity, socialising, enjoying creative hobbies, and having simple moments of stillness. The consequence is weakening relationships, declining fitness, and a growing disconnection from nature and community.

Even our minds are affected. The term 'brain rot' has entered the lexicon to describe the fragmented attention and mental fatigue that follows endless scrolling. Platforms built to deliver constant dopamine hits, such as social media, short-form videos, and even endless news feeds, train our brains to expect instant gratification. The result is a reduced ability to focus intensely, think critically, or even sit with boredom.

The Health Effects of Excessive Screen Time

We already know that too much screen time is not good for us. But we often underestimate how far-reaching the effects can be.

Physical health

- Eye strain, dry eyes, blurred vision, and frequent headaches are common complaints.
- Screen use disrupts sleep by interfering with melatonin production, especially with night-time exposure to blue light.
- A sedentary lifestyle caused by extended sitting is a leading risk factor for obesity, heart disease, and type 2 diabetes.
- Repetitive strain injuries such as carpal tunnel syndrome and tendonitis are increasing.
- Poor posture and muscle weakness are becoming increasingly common even among the young.

Mental health

- Excessive screen time, especially on social media, has been linked to anxiety, depression, and loneliness.
- The curated perfection of others' lives can lead to low self-esteem and negative body image.

- Superficial digital connections often replace deeper, more fulfilling human relationships.
- Shorter attention spans, weaker memory, and reduced learning capacity are all consequences of non-stop digital consumption.
- Sleep disturbances from late-night screen use worsen mental health and impair emotional regulation.

Simple Steps Towards a Digital Detox

The first step to breaking free is recognising there is a problem. The next step is taking small, sustainable steps to make a change.

- **Set boundaries**: Decide on tech-free periods such as mealtimes, an hour before bed, or while exercising. Leave your phone behind for walks. Use apps that track and limit screen time (ironic, yes, but useful).
- **Create tech-free zones**: Make certain areas of your home, like the bedroom or dining table, off-limits to screens. Charge your phone in another room to prevent mindless scrolling before sleep.
- **Mute the noise**: Turn off non-essential notifications. You do not need your phone to summon you every few seconds. Reclaim your attention.
- **Rediscover offline joy**: Make time for hobbies that do not involve screens, such as reading, painting, gardening, baking, music, and movement. Let your hands and senses remember what it is like to create without a touchscreen. Carry a small notebook everywhere jot down and to read your thoughts.
- **Practise mindfulness**: Meditation, yoga, deep breathing – these are not just buzzwords. They retrain your nervous system to slow down, helping reverse the stress patterns of digital overexposure.
- **Protect your sleep**: Establish a soothing pre-sleep routine without screens. Dim the lights, read a physical book, or listen to calming music. Good sleep is one of the most powerful resets for the brain.
- **Seek support when needed**: If you or someone you know feels genuinely stuck, it may be more than just a bad habit. Screen addiction is real, and mental health professionals can offer strategies tailored to your needs.

Putting It into Practice
- Take a short walk each day, leaving your phone behind.
- Pick up a hobby you left behind in childhood that never needed a screen.

Recommended reading

- *Dopamine Detox: A Short Guide to Remove Distractions and Get Your Brain to Do Hard Things* by Thibaut Meurisse

You've Got This

Screen addiction is a predictable outcome of brilliantly engineered devices and platforms designed to capture and hold our attention. But you have the power to reshape your habits. You do not need to go off-grid, just learn to navigate the digital world mindfully, and appreciate the full richness of life.

9

Running on Empty: How to Recognise and Recover from Burnout

'I used to love my job, but now even opening my laptop feels exhausting.' Milan, a 30-year-old software engineer working with a multinational corporation, was passionate about his work. But lately, he feels exhausted. No amount of sleep feels enough, his patience is paper-thin, and even small tasks feel overwhelming. He cannot remember the last time he felt excited about anything.

If any of this sounds familiar, you might be experiencing burnout.

What Is Burnout?

Burnout is much more than tiredness. It is a deep, draining state of physical, emotional, and mental exhaustion caused by prolonged stress. It creeps in quietly as you keep pushing through hectic schedules, balancing home and work, until one day, you hit a brick wall.

Signs of burnout include chronic fatigue (even after rest), lack of motivation for things you used to enjoy, increased irritability, trouble focusing, frequent aches and pains, feeling emotionally detached from work or people, and a general sense of hopelessness that probes the question, 'What's the point?'

Although burnout is not classified as a standalone medical condition, it is widely recognised as a workplace-related syndrome. Its impact on both mental and physical health is real and serious.

Burnout is common, but with the right strategies, you can prevent it, detect it early, or recover if you are already deep in it.

How to Prevent Burnout

Set work boundaries that actually hold

Burnout thrives in an 'always-on' culture. If you do not set limits, work will keep creeping into your personal life.
- Define your work hours and stick to them. Shut your laptop when the workday ends. Say no to extra tasks that you do not have the capacity for.
- Take real breaks. Not at your desk. Not while checking Slack.
- Mute notifications after hours. The world will not end.

Give your brain and body a breather

Pushing through exhaustion will not get you ahead; it will just make you crash.
- Take micro-breaks: stretch, walk, breathe, look at some trees.
- Move daily: yoga, a walk, a game of pickleball, everything counts.
- Prioritise sleep: cut screen time before bed, create a calming routine.

Protect your mental bandwidth

Your brain is not a machine; stop treating it like one.
- Mute unnecessary WhatsApp groups. Turn off non-urgent alerts.
- Unfollow content that leaves you feeling anxious or inadequate.
- Schedule joy: hobbies, music, a chai break, or doing absolutely nothing.

Manage stress before it manages you

Stress is part of life. Chronic stress does not have to be.
- Try meditation, journalling, deep breathing, or a real conversation.
- Do something with your hands: cook, garden, sketch, build.
- Laugh. Watch silly videos. Share memes. Call that hilarious friend.

Burnt Out Already? Here Is How to Recover

Pause and acknowledge it

Accept that you are burnt out. This is not just you being lazy or in a bad mood. Recognise the red flags your body and mind

are showing you. Instead of pushing harder, take a step back and ask:
- What is draining me the most?
- What can I pause or delegate?
- What do I actually need right now?

Prioritise rest and recovery
- Take time off, if possible. Even a few days off can support your mental health and reset your system.
- Allow yourself to do nothing. Rest is not 'wasting time', and you do not always have to be productive.
- Slow down your schedule. Reduce commitments, and say no to unnecessary tasks.

Rebuild energy with small wins
- When you are burnt out, even basic tasks can feel overwhelming. Instead of trying to 'fix everything', focus on small, manageable steps. Start with one tiny habit such as a 10-minute walk, reading for fun, or going to bed 30 minutes earlier.
- Break big tasks into smaller chunks. Instead of 'finish filing column', break it into 'do research', 'note down important points', 'write the first draft', and 'edit'.
- Celebrate small wins. Even checking something off your to-do list (even if it is 'make the to-do list') counts.

Seek support

Burnout thrives in isolation. You do not have to fix it alone. Support could come from talking to someone; for example, emotional support from friends and family, practical support by delegating tasks, or professional support from a therapist or coach.

Putting It into Practice

- Identify one area where you are overextending yourself. Set a boundary there and stick to it.
- Prioritise one recovery step today. It could be extra rest, a joyful activity, or a screen break. Remember, rest is productive.

Recommended reading

- *Burnout: The Secret to Unlocking the Stress Cycle* by Emily Nagoski and Amelia Nagoski

You've Got This

Burnout does not mean you are weak or incapable. It means you have been running on empty for too long. With small, steady steps, you can refill your tank and regain your energy and enthusiasm.

10

Laughter, Ritual, Belonging: The Science of Social Wellness

The morning laughter clubs echoing through the local park, the jovial buzz of kitty parties, the soothing rhythm of weekly group chants or devotional bhajans – on the surface, these might seem like casual social meetups. But look closer, and you will notice something more profound – a thread of community woven tightly into the fabric of well-being.

In my residential complex, we often joke that the senior citizens have a more active social calendar than the younger families. They are part of a WhatsApp group called 'Ammazaans' (a play on the Amazon rainforest), and they are always having lunch potlucks, cultural programmes, crocheting for charity, and birthday celebrations. Their lives are punctuated with purpose, companionship, and a constant sense of belonging.

I recently watched a thought-provoking video on Instagram. The speaker said: 'It takes a village, but you also need to be part of the village and contribute back.' That sentiment captures the essence of community. It is not just something we receive; it is something we take part in, give back to, and nurture.

The Evolutionary Need for Connection

Our need to connect has been present since ancient times. For most of human history, our survival relied on others. Tribes offered protection, shared resources, and emotional support. Even today, our nervous systems carry that legacy. The same brain regions that register physical pain are activated during social rejection. That is why loneliness does not just feel bad; it hurts.

The Science of Social Connection

It is a well-established scientific fact that humans are social creatures. Studies across various disciplines have consistently demonstrated the profound impact of social relationships on physical and mental health.

Physiological impact

Social connection triggers the release of oxytocin, often called the 'love hormone', which reduces stress, lowers blood pressure, and strengthens the immune system. Conversely, social isolation activates the hypothalamic–pituitary–adrenal (HPA) axis, leading to increased cortisol levels, chronic inflammation, and impaired immune function. Research indicates that strong social ties are associated with a reduced risk of cardiovascular disease, stroke, certain cancers,[10] and overall mortality.[11]

One of the most famous examples of this comes from the Roseto Effect, a study of a small Italian–American community in Pennsylvania.[12] It was found that, despite poor diets and high smoking rates, the town's residents had significantly lower heart disease rates than neighbouring areas. Researchers traced this unexpected benefit to their tight social bonds – shared meals, multigenerational households, and a culture of mutual support.

Mental well-being

Supportive relationships protect us against stress, anxiety, and depression. A sense of belonging builds resilience and helps us weather life's challenges. Knowing someone has your back can be just as healing as any supplement or therapy.

Longevity

The research is sobering. Loneliness is as harmful to health as smoking 15 cigarettes a day.[13] People with strong social networks tend to live longer, healthier lives. Social isolation, on the other hand, is a major risk factor for chronic illness and early death.

The Loneliness Epidemic

Despite living in an era of hyper-connectivity, many feel lonelier than ever. Long work hours, urban lifestyles, and endless digital scrolling have eroded face-to-face relationships. Social media might keep us updated, but a like or emoji cannot replace genuine laughter, eye contact, or a reassuring touch on the shoulder. We are more 'connected' than ever, and yet, increasingly isolated.

The Power of Community

Strong communities do more than offer companionship. They provide emotional safety nets, share resources, and cultivate a sense of purpose. During the COVID-19 pandemic, this became abundantly clear. Neighbours delivered groceries to the elders. Mental health check-ins were organised via video calls for isolated individuals. Entire apartment complexes came together in support of each other.

As the saying goes, a good neighbour can be better than a distant relative.

Practical Ways to Reconnect

If this aspect of life has been quietly slipping through the cracks, here are some practical, realistic steps to bring connection back into focus:

- **Prioritise real connection**: Even with a packed schedule, find time for people who matter. A call, a meal, a walk, even brief, meaningful interactions count.
- **Join a group or cause**: Look for clubs, cultural circles, walking groups, or volunteer initiatives. Shared interests create natural bonding opportunities.
- **Give back**: Community is not just about receiving. Offer help, share knowledge, and celebrate others' wins. Be the support you would want to receive.
- **Embrace vulnerability**: Genuine connection requires honesty. Let people in, share your joys and struggles, and ask for help when needed.
- **Value micro-connections**: Not everyone thrives in large groups, and that is okay. Even small interactions such as chatting with a neighbour, greeting a shopkeeper, or engaging in a brief conversation with a co-worker can contribute to a sense of belonging.

Putting It into Practice

Building and maintaining meaningful connections is a vital component of your health blueprint. Start small. Schedule a weekly coffee meeting with a friend, join a local walking group, or volunteer at the local school. Remember, connection is a two-way street. Be present, listen actively, and offer support to others.

You've Got This

You are not alone on this journey. We all crave connection, and we all benefit from it. By consciously cultivating our social relationships, we not only improve our own well-being but also contribute to the health of our community.

Part VIII

Living Long, Living Well

1. Live Like a Centenarian: Blue Zones' Rules
2. Steady Steps: How to Prevent Falls
3. Building Stronger Bones and Muscles for Life
4. Your Brain's Not Done Yet: Outsmarting Cognitive Decline

1

Live Like a Centenarian: Blue Zones' Rules

The Blue Zones are longevity hotspots around the world where people live significantly longer and healthier lives, often reaching 100 years or more. Think Okinawa (Japan), Sardinia (Italy), Nicoya (Costa Rica), Icaria (Greece), and Loma Linda (California). They have been studied to identify lifestyle habits that contribute to longevity. These folks are not chasing fads or guzzling kale smoothies; they just live differently. Learn their secrets and make small tweaks to your current routine for a longer, better life.

Habits You Can Adopt

Eat a plant-forward diet

- **Blue Zone habit**: Their diets are 90–95 per cent plant-based, centred around vegetables, legumes (beans, lentils), whole grains, and nuts. Meat is eaten sparingly, often as a side or on special occasions.
- **How to implement**: Shift your meals towards plant-based options. If you have a meat-heavy diet, try going vegetarian twice a week. Replace processed snacks with nuts or fruit. Make beans a staple in your diet – whether as curries, salads, soups, sundal (a variety of cooked beans with tadka), hummus, etc. Limit UPFs and red meat.

Move naturally

- **Blue Zone habit**: People in Blue Zones do not rely on gyms or CrossFit workouts. Instead, they keep active through everyday activities like gardening, walking, or manual labour.

- **How to implement**: Sitting for long hours at a desk job? Incorporate more natural movement into your routine. Walk or cycle instead of driving short distances, take the stairs instead of the elevator, or start a small garden on your balcony or in your community. Aim for at least 30 minutes of low-intensity activity most days.

Stop before you are stuffed

- **Blue Zone habit**: Most of these populations often practise unconscious caloric restriction. Okinawans follow 'Hara Hachi Bu', eating until they are 80 per cent full. Meals are usually served in smaller portions, and snacking is uncommon.
- **How to implement**: Use smaller plates to naturally limit portion sizes. Eat slowly to notice fullness and prevent late-night munchies.

Prioritise social connections

- **Blue Zone habit**: Strong family and community bonds are common. People live with or near loved ones, maintain lifelong friendships, and participate in social groups.
- **How to implement**: Spend time building relationships – call a friend, join a club or group based on a shared interest, or host regular dinners with family or neighbours. Loneliness can harm our health, so build your 'tribe'.

Find your purpose

- **Blue Zone habit**: Having a sense of purpose, or 'ikigai' (Okinawa) or 'plan de vida' (Nicoya), guides daily life and lowers stress.
- **How to implement**: Reflect on what motivates you, whether it is a hobby, volunteering, or a career goal, and dedicate time to it. Even small daily goals (e.g., helping someone) can improve well-being.

Manage your stress

- **Blue Zone habit**: They follow routines to reduce stress, such as napping (Icaria), praying (Loma Linda), or sharing tea with friends (Okinawa).

- **How to implement**: Build a stress-relief routine as part of your day – meditate for 10 minutes, take a short walk, or practise deep breathing. Visit your place of worship and pray if that is something you do. Limit screen time, especially before bed.

Drink in moderation or not at all

- **Blue Zone habit**: Many people enjoy small amounts of wine (e.g., Sardinia's Cannonau) with meals and friends, but excessive drinking is rare.
- **How to implement**: If you drink, limit it to one to two glasses of wine with dinner, occasionally, ideally with company. Avoid binge drinking.

Belong to a faith or spiritual community

- **Blue Zone habit**: Most centenarians are part of a faith or community group that they regularly attend for support and purpose.
- **How to implement**: Find a spiritual practice or community that resonates with you, whether religious, secular (such as a meditation group), or musical (like bhajan or chanting groups), and participate regularly.

Put family first

- **Blue Zone habit**: Multigenerational living is common, with elders looked after and younger generations supported.
- **How to implement**: Strengthen family bonds by spending quality time with parents, children, or siblings, and consider involving grandparents in daily life if possible.

Putting It into Practice

- **Today**: Replace one processed snack with a handful of nuts or a piece of fruit.
- **This week**: Plan a walk with friends or family instead of hanging out at a cafe.
- **This month**: Try cooking a Blue Zone-inspired meal, such as sweet potatoes with beans, tofu, and a dressing or sauce, and invite someone to share it.

Add these habits gradually and make them a part of your lifestyle.

You've Got This

You do not have to rely on flashy biohacks or expensive supplements – just simple, everyday habits that add up over time. Folks living in Blue Zones have stayed away from modern traps like processed food or endless scrolling. Start small, stay consistent, and you will not only live longer but also enjoy a better quality of life.

2

Steady Steps: How to Prevent Falls

My grandmother remained independent well into her 70s and 80s, helping with kitchen chores, taking daily walks, and attending family events. She suffered a fall that resulted in a fractured femur neck, followed by surgery and a slow, painful recovery from which she never fully regained her strength or health. She passed away soon afterwards.

Not all accidents end in disaster, but they often lessen life's brightness – reducing confidence, limiting outings, and increasing isolation. In India, seniors tripping, slipping, or falling remains a major concern. However, they are not unavoidable. Through small, deliberate changes, we can safeguard our bodies, increase strength, prolong our physical independence, and extend our years. We have the power to intentionally lay the groundwork for a longer, healthier life.

The Silent Risk We Cannot Ignore

In the Blue Zones, the longevity hotspots of the world like Okinawa and Sardinia, where people routinely live past 100, accidents such as falling are rare. Because movement is woven into their days, not as Zumba classes but as a natural rhythm, such as tending gardens and walking hilly paths. Contrast that with our modern lives, where a third of older adults – over 14 million in the US alone – deal with accidental falls each year. In India, nearly 31 per cent of people over 60 experience a fall.[1]

These numbers are more than just statistics; they serve as warning signs. Falls lead to hospital stays and emergency visits, robbing people of 38 million healthy years worldwide.[2]

The actual cost of a fall is in what comes afterwards: losing confidence in one's own body, fearing a walk to the store, feeling isolated when stairs seem like hurdles. However, science shows us this is not something we have to accept. From the Blue Zones to the latest research, we know falls can be prevented. Let us understand how.

Building Strength

Strength is your first line of defence. A study in India found that poor balance triples fall risk.[3] But the fix is within reach. In Icaria, Greece, centenarians climb rocky trails without hesitation, their legs and core strengthened by decades of climbing. Exercises like Tai Chi can cut fall risk by 50 per cent, while simple leg lifts or chair squats help rebuild stability. Set aside 20 minutes a few times a week for simple exercises as part of your daily routine. You can also integrate some movement into your routine like brushing your teeth while balancing on one leg or standing up from a chair without using your hands. Strength training in the gym is not just for the young. Even people over 60 can benefit greatly from basic compound exercises. Consider working with a certified coach who specialises in training seniors. Start small, progress gradually, and your body will thank you.

Make Home a Safe Space

Your home should be a safe space, not a hazard. Remove loose rugs, uneven flooring, and dim lighting. Keep rooms brightly lit, as vision loss doubles the risk of falls. Secure rugs, if using, with double-sided tape, install grab bars near the toilet, and use anti-skid tiles in the bathroom. Clear clutter, such as stray wires or stacks of books, that could cause tripping. Research ways to make your home fall-proof, and ask a family member or neighbour for help. If you live with elderly loved ones, these simple steps can help prevent serious trouble.

Tools and Senses

Choosing the right gear matters. Swap slippery socks for shoes with grips. Falls often start with a skid. Do not feel ashamed about using a cane or a walker. Technology can help too – wearable alarms that can detect a fall and call for help. Make sure to get regular eye and ear check-ups. Blurry eyesight or muffled sounds can throw you off balance, but both are fixable. In India, where 51 per cent of older adults manage multiple health conditions, a quick doctor visit to adjust medications (dizziness is a common side effect) can steady your steps.

Rising After a Fall

Even the steadiest among us might slip someday. That is why knowing how to get up, such as rolling to your side or crawling to a chair, matters. Practising these habits builds muscle memory, which can prevent adverse consequences. You can find several exercises online on how to 'fall right', and if you practise them often enough, these reflexes will activate and help you if you ever fall.

Putting It into Practice

You do not have to overhaul your entire life to prevent falls. It is about gradually developing habits that last. Try standing on one leg while the kettle boils. Swap a dim bulb for a bright one. Take a walk with a friend.

You've Got This

Every step you take, no matter how small, strengthens your body and spirit. By building strength and preventing falls, you create a life where each day feels freer and bolder. Embrace the journey. You have the power to keep moving forward, safely.

3

Building Stronger Bones and Muscles for Life

One in three women over 50 will face an osteoporotic fracture, according to the International Osteoporosis Foundation. This serves as a sobering reminder that ageing can quietly weaken our body's foundation. Two age-related conditions, sarcopenia and osteoporosis, contribute significantly to this decline, impairing mobility, increasing injury risks, and threatening independence. However, these are not unavoidable outcomes. Through targeted nutrition, regular exercise, and smart lifestyle choices, we can strengthen our bodies and age with strength, stability, and confidence.

Understanding Sarcopenia and Osteoporosis

Sarcopenia, the gradual loss of muscle mass, strength, and function, often begins in the 40s and speeds up after 60, raising the risks of falls, fractures, metabolic problems, and even death. Osteoporosis, characterised by low bone density and deteriorating bone tissue, makes bones brittle and more likely to fracture. Both conditions often develop silently, only becoming apparent after a fall or fracture. Osteoporosis is diagnosed with a DEXA scan, while sarcopenia is assessed by measuring muscle mass, strength (like grip strength), and performance (such as walking speed).

Gender Differences in Sarcopenia and Osteoporosis

Men and women experience sarcopenia and osteoporosis differently because of hormonal, physiological, and lifestyle factors.

In women, osteoporosis risk increases after menopause as falling oestrogen accelerates loss of bone density. As noted, one in three women over 50 will face an osteoporotic fracture globally.

Sarcopenia also affects women more post-menopause, as the decline in oestrogen accelerates muscle loss. Women's lower baseline muscle mass increases the functional impact, leading to earlier fatigue, reduced mobility, and greater frailty. Contributing factors include lower participation in resistance training and inadequate protein intake.

In men, sarcopenia often appears earlier and more noticeably, caused by a gradual decline in testosterone that weakens muscle mass and bone density. Although men start with higher muscle and bone mass, they might not realise the gradual loss until it affects daily activities or causes injury.

The Role of Muscle in Healthy Ageing

Muscles do more than just power movement or flex for appearance. They are vital for metabolic health, regulating blood glucose, and maintaining bone strength. Muscle mass acts as a reservoir for amino acids and helps support balance and mobility. During movement, muscles apply mechanical force on bones, stimulating bone growth and emphasising the deep connection between these systems.[4] This synergy is key to ageing with resilience.

The Importance of Protein

Protein intake is the most effective nutritional defence against sarcopenia and supports bone health. As we age, our bodies become less efficient at synthesising muscle protein. To counteract this, older adults require higher protein intake compared to younger adults. The general recommendation is 1.2 to 1.5 g/kg of body weight daily for healthy older adults. Higher intakes (up to 2 g/kg) may benefit active individuals, those recovering from illness, or those with diagnosed sarcopenia. The quality of protein is also important. Prioritise complete proteins such as lean meats, dairy, eggs, soy, and quinoa, or ensure you eat a diverse range of plant-based foods to obtain all the essential amino acids in a day.

The Importance of Exercise

Resistance training is the most effective way to slow or reverse sarcopenia.[5] Exercises with weights, resistance bands, or body weight stimulate muscle growth and strength. Resistance training also benefits bone density by activating osteoblasts, the cells responsible for bone formation. For bone health, weight-bearing and impact-loading activities like walking, stair climbing, or strength training are most beneficial.[6] The synergy between exercise and protein is powerful: muscles respond better to protein after exercise, making post-workout nutrition especially effective.[7]

The Importance of Other Nutritional Factors

While protein takes centre stage, supportive nutrients are essential too:
- **Vitamin D**: Vital for both bone health and muscle function. Low levels are linked to higher rates of falls, fractures, and muscle weakness
- **Calcium and magnesium**: Essential for bone mineralisation
- **Vitamin K2**: Helps guide calcium into bones and away from arteries
- **Omega-3s**: May help preserve muscle mass and reduce inflammation
- **Creatine**: Enhances muscle strength and lean mass in older adults when paired with resistance training (to be taken after consulting your doctor)

Putting It into Practice

- Aim for 1.2–1.5 g/kg body weight daily (e.g., eggs, soy, lean meats).
- Do resistance exercises (weights, bands) three times a week.
- Take your vitamin D, calcium, and omega-3s.
- Test grip strength or gait speed; schedule DEXA scans.

You've Got This

Ageing is an opportunity to thrive. By combining smart nutrition, regular exercise, and healthy lifestyle choices, you can protect yourself from the silent threats of sarcopenia and osteoporosis. Every protein-rich meal, every weight lifted, every mindful step forward is a step towards a confident future. Your body is your lifelong ally – empower it to live stronger, longer.

4

Your Brain's Not Done Yet: Outsmarting Cognitive Decline

The world is feeding you a lie. Shuffling seniors forgetting PINs, searching for glasses perched on their heads, or blanking on their neighbour's name – these are lazy stereotypes meant to make you accept cognitive decline as inevitable. Do not buy into it. Your brain is a powerhouse, capable of rewiring itself into your eighties and beyond. While mental health steals the spotlight, cognitive health – your memory, focus, and problem-solving skills – is an equally important component you cannot ignore. Ready to take control? Here is how to boost your brain with science and keep it sharp for life.

Cognitive Reserve: Your Brain's Backup Plan

Think of your brain as a Swiss Army knife, equipped with a tool for every situation. That is cognitive reserve, your brain's knack for avoiding age-related damage like a skilled boxer. It is your mind's ability to withstand damage and keep working at full speed.

Research in *The Lancet Neurology* drops a truth bomb – some people's brains stay sharp despite having Alzheimer's disease because they built up extra mental strength over their lifetime.[8] Some even die with plaque-filled brains but show no symptoms in life, because their cognitive reserve is a fortress, easily keeping off all damage.

Cognitive reserve is not just for IIT-IIM graduates (though education boosts neural connections). It is about keeping your brain active and engaged with new challenges. Here is how to build it:

- **Flex your mind**: Jobs that demand complex problem-solving – think engineers, strategists, or sharp entrepreneurs – boost your cognitive resilience.
- **Have fun hobbies**: Reading Tolstoy, shredding guitar solos (or creating Hindustani music taans), or playing chess builds new neural pathways.
- **Get social**: Deep conversations, heated debates, or interacting with friends challenge your brain to balance memory, empathy, and quick thinking.
- **Never stop learning**: Pick up coding, learn Italian, or geek out on astrophysics. Every new skill is a deposit in your cognitive bank.

A *JAMA Neurology* study found that each additional brain-stimulating activity you add to your routine reduces dementia risk by about 17 per cent. Combine those activities, and you are building a cognitive fortress.[9]

The Heart–Brain Connection

Your brain is a diva, demanding a VIP delivery of oxygen and nutrients to keep the show going. Skimp on vascular health, and your neurons throw a fit. A study showed that middle-aged adults who had poorer cardiovascular fitness tended to have smaller brains about 20 years later.[10] Staying fit in midlife is important to protect the brain and keep it healthier as we age.

Here is how to keep the blood flowing:
- **Blood pressure**: High blood pressure is a stealthy assassin, damaging tiny brain vessels and increasing the risk of vascular dementia. Keep it under control.
- **Get moving**: Exercise releases brain-derived neurotrophic factor (BDNF), a fertiliser for neurons that boosts learning and memory. A daily brisk walk works wonders.
- **Sugar control**: Chronic high blood sugar damages your brain's delicate vessels, sparking inflammation and cognitive haze. Keep it under check.
- **Sleep like you mean it**: Deep sleep activates your brain's glymphatic system, the clean-up crew that flushes out harmful waste like beta-amyloid, a key player in Alzheimer's.

The Mediterranean diet, with its olive oil, fish, and vegetables, helps keep your vascular system healthy, keeping your brain working at its best.

Neuroinflammation: Your Brain's Silent Enemy

Chronic inflammation is your brain's nemesis. *Frontiers in Ageing Neuroscience* ties inflammatory markers to faster cognitive decline.[11] Some triggers are out of your hands, but there is a lot you can control.

- **Diet**: Avoid UPFs and omega-6-heavy oils. Instead, load up on antioxidant-rich foods like colourful fruits and veggies, salmon, and polyphenol-rich greens.
- **Exercise**: Regular exercise reduces inflammatory markers like IL-6, which mess with your neurons.
- **Stress**: Chronic cortisol spikes from stress are like setting fire to your neurons. Find your de-stressors like yoga, kickboxing, or dancing.
- **Sleep**: If you don't get enough sleep, inflammatory cytokines sneak past your blood–brain barrier. Give sleep the importance it deserves.
- **Gut health**: Your gut and brain are in constant touch. A healthy microbiome cuts inflammatory chatter that clouds cognition.

Putting It into Practice

Here is the resilient brain's playbook:

- **Never stop learning**: Learn a new instrument, dive into philosophy, or master Brazilian jiu-jitsu. Challenge multiple brain domains for maximum gains.
- **Sleep like it is your superpower**: Lock in seven to eight hours of deep rest. Get snoring and insomnia fixed because untreated sleep issues are cognitive poison.
- **Move with purpose**: 30 minutes of brisk walking 5 days a week slashes the risk of mental decline. Toss in weights or yoga for extra points.
- **Eat like your brain's watching**: Prioritise whole foods, colourful produce, and healthy fats.
- **Stay curious**: Keep asking questions, exploring, and pushing your limits. A curious mind is a resilient mind.

Recommended reading

- *The Brain That Changes Itself* by Norman Doidge

You've Got This

Cognitive decline is a gradual process that begins in your 30s or 40s, and if you don't take any action, it can dull your mental sharpness by the time you turn 70. Your brain's plasticity is your secret weapon, ready to forge new connections. But it is up to you to nurture it with exercise, sleep, wholesome food, and a life that keeps you always curious. So, what is the plan? Drift towards a foggy future or take control and stay endlessly curious? Your neurons are waiting for their marching orders.

Acknowledgements

I want to begin by thanking all the teachers and professors from school, medical college, and beyond, who encouraged and nurtured my curiosity in science. When, in third grade, my science teacher wrote, 'Well done, my budding scientist!', something shifted in me, and it set me on this path.

My late father, R. Viswanathan, who became deeply committed to his health in his later years, would have loved to see me writing a book that simplifies health for everyone.

My music guru, Shri Mahesh Kale, whose guidance has enriched not only my music but also the way I approach life and work, and step beyond my comfort zones.

My long-time friend Krish Ashok, who got me started on sharing more science-backed health content on social media, a step that laid the groundwork for this book.

All my followers on Instagram and X, and the early followers of my blog, who have taken the time to view and engage with my content, share their experiences, and help me understand the common health struggles people face.

My editor, Chirag Thakkar, with whom my paths have crossed thrice thus far. He pursued and pushed me to write this book on health. I value our quiet understanding of each other that has helped us bring this beautiful book to reality.

My sister, Nivedita, who went from couch to running full marathons around the world with sheer grit and dedication.

My husband, Sumanth, whose determination to run ultramarathons in places where few dare to go, and disciplined approach to health, inspires everyone around him.

My son, Atri, whose very presence fills my life with purpose and fulfilment.

And finally, my dog, Ida. Cuddling with her is my number-one stress buster, absolutely vital for keeping my sanity when deadlines are looming.

Notes

PART I The Foundations

1. 'Vidya Balan's Weight-Loss Journey, Her Diet and a Medical Condition', The Free Press Journal, 4 December 2024, YouTube, https://www.youtube.com/watch?v=wKTKUPv7-BA.
2. Matej Mikulic, 'Dietary Supplements with Largest Increase in Usage due to COVID-19 Among U.S. Adults as of August 2020', Statista, 19 October 2020, https://www.statista.com/statistics/1180337/top-dietary-supplement-usage-growth-due-to-covid-us-adults/?srsltid=AfmBOoow3uwioeGvShelpygig9o80qsNPiCX6pSi_k2g2AFg3dU707Wp.
3. A.A. Prather et al., 'Negative Affective Responses to a Speech Task Predict Changes in Interleukin (IL)-6', *Sleep* 38, no. 9 (2015): 1355–1363, https://doi.org/10.5665/sleep.4968.
5. S.M. Chastin et al., 'Effects of Regular Physical Activity on the Immune System, Vaccination and Risk of Community-Acquired Infectious Disease in the General Population: Systematic Review and Meta-Analysis', *Sports Medicine* 51, no. 8 (2021): 1673–1686, https://doi.org/10.1007/s40279-021-01466-1.
6. S.C. Segerstrom and G.E. Miller, 'Psychological Stress and the Human Immune System: A Meta-Analytic Study of 30 Years of Inquiry', *Psychoneuroendocrinology* 114 (2020): 104620, https://doi.org/10.1016/j.psyneuen.2020.104620.
7. D.S. Black and G.M. Slavich, 'Mindfulness Meditation and the Immune System: A Systematic Review of Randomized Controlled Trials', *Journal of Behavioral Medicine* 41, no. 4 (2018): 485–500, https://doi.org/10.1007/s10865-018-9917-0.
8. B.N. Uchino et al., 'Social Relationships and Immune Function: A Meta-Analysis', *Psychosomatic Medicine* 81, no. 2 (2019): 133–141, https://doi.org/10.1097/PSY.0000000000000661.
9. Zheng Yawei et al., 'The Gut Microbiome and the Immune System', *Nature Reviews Immunology* 18, no.5 (2018): 323–336.
10. 'No Level of Alcohol Consumption Is Safe for Our Health', World Health Organization, 4 January 2023, https://www.who.int/europe/news/item/04-01-2023-no-level-of-alcohol-consumption-is-safe-for-our-health.

11 PTI, '38 per cent of Indians Suffer from Non-Alcoholic Fatty Liver Disease: Report', *Economic Times*, 2 August 2023, https://economictimes.indiatimes.com/magazines/panache/38-per-cent-of-indians-suffer-from-non-alcoholic-fatty-liver-disease-report/articleshow/102358315.cms.

12 'Get Checked Before 30: Dr Naresh Trehan Warns of Heart Risks Post-Covid Recover', *India Today*, 17 February 2025, https://www.indiatoday.in/india/story/heart-attack-young-people-covid-diabetes-family-history-health-checkup-medanta-hospital-dr-naresh-trehan-2681457-2025-02-17.

PART II Food, Fad, and Fiction

1 Frederick J. Stare and Margaret McWilliams, *Nutrition for Good Health: Eating Less and Living Longer!* (1982).

2 J. Gunter, 'How Much Water Do You Actually Need a Day?' TED, May 2021, https://www.ted.com/talks/body_stuff_with_dr_jen_gunter_how_much_water_do_you_actually_need_a_day.

3 J. Trommelen et al., 'The Anabolic Response to Protein Ingestion During Recovery from Exercise Has No Upper Limit in Magnitude and Duration In Vivo in Humans', *Cell Reports Medicine* 4, no. 12 (2023), https://pubmed.ncbi.nlm.nih.gov/38118410/.

4 'Ayushmann Khurrana's Life Hacks on Confidence, Spirituality & Fitness', BeerBiceps, 7 November 2019, YouTube, 11:36, https://www.youtube.com/watch?v=d3R2-nW065U&t=692s.

5 J. Antonio et al., 'A High Protein Diet Has No Harmful Effects: A One-Year Crossover Study in Resistance-Trained Males', *Journal of Nutrition and Metabolism* (2016), https://pubmed.ncbi.nlm.nih.gov/27807480/.

6 L. Brown et al., 'Cholesterol-Lowering Effects of Dietary Fiber: A Meta-analysis', *The American Journal of Clinical Nutrition* 69, no. 1 (1999): 30–42.

7 I.S. Waddell and C. Orfila, 'Dietary Fiber in the Prevention of Obesity and Obesity-related Chronic Diseases: From Epidemiological Evidence to Potential Molecular Mechanisms', *Critical Reviews in Food Science and Nutrition* 63, no. 27 (2022): 8752–8767.

8 C. Sidharthan, 'The Role of Fiber in Preventing Chronic Disease', *News Medical*, 17 March 2025, https://www.news-medical.net/health/The-Role-of-Fiber-in-Preventing-Chronic-Disease.aspx.

9 Kerri M. Gillespie et al., 'The Impact of Free Sugar on Human Health – A Narrative Review', *Nutrients* 15, no. 4 (2023): 889.

10 *Guideline: Sugars Intake for Adults and Children* (Geneva: World Health Organization, 2015), https://www.who.int/publications/i/item/9789241549028.

11 A.S. Christensen et al.,'Effect of Fruit Restriction on Glycemic Control in Patients with Type 2 Diabetes – A Randomized Trial', *Nutrition Journal* 12 (2013): 29, https://nutritionj.biomedcentral.com/articles/10.1186/1475-2891-12-29.
12 Marcin Barański et al., 'Higher Antioxidant and Lower Cadmium Concentrations and Lower Incidence of Pesticide Residues in Organically Grown Crops: A Systematic Literature Review and Meta-Analyses', *The British Journal of Nutrition* 112, no. 5, (2014): 794–811.
13 Ibid.
14 *National Family Health Survey (NFHS-5), 2019–2021: India Report* (International Institute for Population Sciences (IIPS) and ICF, 2021), https://www.dhsprogram.com/pubs/pdf/FR375/FR375.pdf.
15 Harriet Rumgay et al., 'Global Burden of Cancer in 2020 Attributable to Alcohol Consumption: A Population-based Study', *The Lancet Oncology* 22, no. 8 (2021): 1071-1080.
16 'No Level of Alcohol Consumption Is Safe for Our Health', World Health Organization, 4 January 2023, https://www.who.int/europe/news/item/04-01-2023-no-level-of-alcohol-consumption-is-safe-for-our-health.
17 S. Weiskirchen and R. Weiskirchen, 'Resveratrol: How Much Wine Do You Have to Drink to Stay Healthy?', *Advances in Nutrition* 7, no. 4 (2016): 706–718.

PART III Built to Move

1 *WHO Guidelines on Physical Activity and Sedentary Behaviour* (Geneva: World Health Organization, 2020), https://www.who.int/publications/i/item/9789240015128.
2 Stamatina Iliodromiti et al., 'Should Physical Activity Recommendations for South Asian Adults Be Ethnicity-Specific? Evidence from a Cross-Sectional Study of South Asian and White European Men and Women', *PLOS One* 11, no. 8 (2016).
3 D.P. Bailey, 'Breaking Up Prolonged Sitting with Light-Intensity Walking Improves Postprandial Glycemia, But Breaking Up Sitting with Standing Does Not', *Journal of Science and Medicine in Sport* 18, no. 3 (2015): 294–298, https://pubmed.ncbi.nlm.nih.gov/24704421/.
4 Hamza Ali, 'Why Your Chair Might Be Killing You', CNBC, 18 August 2014, https://www.cnbc.com/2014/08/18/why-your-chair-might-be-killing-you.html.
5 R.M. Anjana et al., 'Physical Activity and Inactivity Patterns in India – Results from the ICMR-INDIAB Study (Phase-1) [ICMR-INDIAB-5]', *The International Journal of Behavioral Nutrition and Physical Activity* 11, no. 26 (2014).

6   E.M. Murtagh et al., 'Walking: The First Steps in Cardiovascular Disease Prevention', *Current Opinion in Cardiology* 25, no. 5 (2010): 490–496.
7   Harvard Health Publishing, 'More Evidence That Exercise Can Boost Mood', *Harvard Health Blog*, 10 March 2022, https://www.health.harvard.edu/mind-and-mood/more-evidence-that-exercise-can-boost-mood.
8   E.A. Krall and B. Dawson-Hughes, 'Walking Is Related to Bone Density and Rates of Bone Loss', *The American Journal of Medicine* 96, no. 1 (1994): 20–26.
9   Harvard Health Publishing, '5 Surprising Benefits of Walking', *Harvard Health Blog*, 7 December 2023, https://www.health.harvard.edu/staying-healthy/5-surprising-benefits-of-walking.
10 A.J. Buffey et al., 'The Acute Effects of Interrupting Prolonged Sitting Time in Adults with Standing and Light-Intensity Walking on Biomarkers of Cardiometabolic Health in Adults: A Systematic Review and Meta-Analysis', *Sports Medicine* 52, no. 8 (2022): 1765–1787.
11 Calorie Calculator, https://www.calculator.net/calorie-calculator.html.

PART IV Your Home, Your Health

1   B. Bekkar et al., 'Association of Air Pollution and Heat Exposure with Preterm Birth, Low Birth Weight, and Stillbirth in the US: A Systematic Review', *JAMA Network Open* 3, no. 6 (2020).
2   C.G. Zundel et al., 'Air Pollution, Depressive and Anxiety Disorders, and Brain Effects: A Systematic Review', *Neurotoxicology* 93 (2022): 272–300, https://doi.org/10.1016/j.neuro.2022.10.011
3   S. Shaw et al., 'Indoor Air Pollution and Cognitive Function Among Older Adults in India: A Multiple Mediation Approach Through Depression and Sleep Disorders', *BMC Geriatrics* 24, no. 81 (2024), https://doi.org/10.1186/s12877-024-04662-6.
4   Energy Policy Institute, University of Chicago, *India Fact Sheet: Air Quality Life Index* (Chicago: University of Chicago, 2021), https://aqli.epic.uchicago.edu/wp-content/uploads/2021/08/IndiaFactSheet_update-.pdf.
5   M.F. Naujokas et al., 'The Broad Scope of Health Effects from Chronic Arsenic Exposure: Update on a Worldwide Public Health Problem', *Environmental Health Perspectives* 121, no. 3 (2013): 295–302.
6   E. Tookmanian, 'Two Studies on Disinfection Byproducts in Drinking Water and Cancer Risk', National Cancer Institute, 31 May 2022, https://dceg.cancer.gov/news-events/news/2022/disinfection-byproducts-drinking-water.

7   L.A. Catling et al., 'A Systematic Review of Analytical Observational Studies Investigating the Association between Cardiovascular Disease and Drinking Water Hardness', *Journal of Water and Health* 6, no. 4 (2008): 433–442.
8   A.N. Thorndike et al., 'Choice Architecture to Promote Fruit and Vegetable Purchases by Families Participating in the Special Supplemental Programme for Women, Infants, and Children (WIC): Randomized Corner Store Pilot Study', *Public Health Nutrition* 20, no. 7 (2017): 1297–1305.
9   H.A. Leslie et al., 'Discovery and Quantification of Plastic Particle Pollution in Human Blood', *Environment International* 163 (2022): 107199.
10 R. Marfella et al., 'Microplastics and Nanoplastics in Atheromas and Cardiovascular Events', *The New England Journal of Medicine* 390, no. 10 (2024): 900–910, https://pubmed.ncbi.nlm.nih.gov/38446676/.
11 World Wildlife Fund, *No Plastic in Nature: Assessing Plastic Ingestion from Nature to People* (Gland: WWF, 2019).
12 M. Sansano et al., 'Effect of Pretreatments and Air-frying, a Novel Technology, on Acrylamide Generation in Fried Potatoes', *Journal of Food Science* 80, no. 5 (2015): T1120–T1128, https://doi.org/10.1111/1750-3841.12843.
13 'The Inside Story: A Guide to Indoor Air Quality', United States Environmental Protection Agency, https://www.epa.gov/indoor-air-quality-iaq/inside-story-guide-indoor-air-quality.
14 B.E. Cummings and M.S. Waring, 'Potted Plants Do Not Improve Indoor Air Quality: A Review and Analysis of Reported VOC Removal Efficiencies', *Journal of Exposure Science & Environmental Epidemiology* 30 (2020): 253–261, https://doi.org/10.1038/s41370-019-0175-9.
15 L. Øie, H. Stymne, C.A. Boman, and V. Hellstrand, 'Volatile Organic Compounds in Indoor Air: Sources and Control', *Indoor Air* 7, no. 2 (1997): 89–107.
16 Ø Svanes et al., 'Cleaning at Home and at Work in Relation to Lung Function Decline and Airway Obstruction', *American Journal of Respiratory and Critical Care Medicine* 197, no. 9 (2018): 1157–1163.
17 M. Kosuth et al., 'Anthropogenic Contamination of Tap Water, Beer, and Sea Salt', *PLOS One* 13, no. 4 (2018), https://doi.org/10.1371/journal.pone.0194970.

PART V The Hormone Connection

1. S.C. Segerstrom and G.E. Miller, 'Psychological Stress and the Human Immune System: A Meta-Analytic Study of 30 Years of Inquiry', *Psychological Bulletin* 130, no. 4 (2004): 601–630, https://doi.org/10.1037/0033-2909.130.4.601.
2. B.S. McEwen, 'Physiology and Neurobiology of Stress and Adaptation: Central Role of the Brain', *Nature Reviews Neuroscience* 8, no. 3 (2007): 200–210, https://doi.org/10.1038/nrn2087.
3. J.A. Foster et al., 'Stress and the Gut-Brain Axis: Regulation by the Microbiome', *Nature Microbiology* 4, no. 12 (2019): 1958–1968, https://doi.org/10.1038/s41564-019-0551-8.
4. L. Wartofsky and R.A. Dickey, 'The Evidence for a Narrower Thyrotropin Reference Range Is Compelling', *The Journal of Clinical Endocrinology & Metabolism* 90, no. 9 (2005): 5483–5488.
5. T.G. Travison et al., 'A Population-Level Decline in Serum Testosterone Levels in American Men', *Journal of Clinical Endocrinology and Metabolism* 92, no. 1 (2007): 196–202, https://doi.org/10.1210/jc.2006-1375.
6. L.J. Moran et al., 'Lifestyle Changes in Women with Polycystic Ovary Syndrome', *Fertility and Sterility* 96, no. 5 (2011): 1108–1115, https://pmc.ncbi.nlm.nih.gov/articles/PMC6438659/.
7. R.A. Bonnema et al., 'Contraception Choices in Women with Underlying Medical Conditions', *American Family Physician* 82, no. 6 (2010): 621–628.
8. E. Mann et al., 'Cognitive Behavioural Therapy for Menopausal Symptoms (Hot Flushes and Night Sweats) in Women: A Randomised Controlled Trial', *Menopause* 25, no. 5 (2018): 531–538, https://doi.org/10.1097/GME.0000000000001047.
9. J.E. Rossouw, G.L. Anderson, R.J. Lambrecht Prentice et al., 'Risks and Benefits of Estrogen Plus Progestin in Healthy Postmenopausal Women: Principal Results from the Women's Health Initiative Randomized Controlled Trial', *JAMA* 288, no. 3 (2002): 321–333, https://doi.org/10.1001/jama.288.3.321.
10. N. Mishra, V.N. Mishra, and Devanshi, 'Exercise Beyond Menopause: Dos and Don'ts', *Journal of Mid-Life Health* 2, no. 2 (2011): 51–56, https://doi.org/10.4103/0976-7800.92524.

PART VI Sleep: The Missing Superpower

1. Matthew Walker, *Why We Sleep* (London: Penguin, 2018).
2. R. Caliandro et al., 'Social Jetlag and Related Risks for Human Health: A Timely Review', *Nutrients* 13, no. 12 (2021): 4543.
3. M. Wittmann et al., 'Social Jetlag: Misalignment of Biological and Social Time', *Chronobiology International* 23, no. 1–2 (2006): 497–509.

4 H.H.K. Fullagar et al., 'Sleep and Athletic Performance: The Effects of Sleep Loss on Exercise Performance, and Physiological and Cognitive Responses to Exercise', *Sports Medicine* 45, no. 2 (2015): 161–186.

PART VII Mind Matters

1 H. Song et al., 'Stress-related Disorders and Risk of Cardiovascular Disease: Population-based, Sibling Controlled Cohort Study', *BMJ* 365 (2019): l1255.
2 R.I. Holt, M. de Groot, and S.H. Golden, 'Diabetes and Depression', *Current Diabetes Reports* 14, no. 6 (2014): 491.
3 A. Babak, N. Motamedi, S.Z. Mousavi, and N. Ghasemi Darestani, 'Effects of Mindfulness-Based Stress Reduction on Blood Pressure, Mental Health, and Quality of Life in Hypertensive Adult Women: A Randomized Clinical Trial Study', *Journal of Tehran University Heart Center* 17, no. 3 (2022): 127–133.
4 B.R. Fry et al., 'Devaluing Memories of Reward: A Case for Dopamine', *Communications Biology* 8, article no. 161 (2025).
5 P. Tyrer et al., 'Increase in the Prevalence of Health Anxiety in Medical Clinics: Possible Cyberchondria', *International Journal of Social Psychiatry* 65, no. 7–8 (2019): 566–569.
6 Lisa Tams, 'Journalling to Reduce COVID-19 Stress', Michigan State University Extension, 11 November 2020, https://www.canr.msu.edu/news/journalling_to_reduce_stress.
7 C.M. Burton and L.A. King, 'Effects of Written Emotional Disclosure on Physiological and Psychological Functioning in Women with Chronic Disease', *Journal of Health Psychology* 9, no. 3 (2004): 427–440.
8 M.K. Scullin, M.L. Krueger, H.K. Ballard et al., 'The Effects of Bedtime Writing on Difficulty Falling Asleep: A Polysomnographic Study Comparing To-do Lists and Completed Activity Lists', *Journal of Experimental Psychology* 147, no. 1 (2018): 139–146.
9 E.A. Locke and G.P. Latham, 'Building a Practically Useful Theory of Goal Setting and Task Motivation: A 35-year Odyssey', *American Psychologist* 57, no. 9 (2002): 705–717.
10 I. Awoyinka et al., 'Examining the Role of Social Relationships on Health and Health Behaviours in African American Men with Prostate Cancer: A Qualitative Analysis', *Supportive Care in Cancer* 32, no. 3 (2024): 178.
11 J. Holt-Lunstad et al., 'Social Relationships and Mortality Risk: A Meta-analytic Review', *PLOS Medicine* 7, no. 7 (2010).
12 B. Egolf, J. Lasker et al., 'The Roseto Effect: A 50-year Comparison of Mortality Rates', *American Journal of Public Health* 82, no. 8 (1992): 1089–1092.

13. *Our Epidemic of Loneliness and Isolation: The U.S. Surgeon General's Advisory on the Healing Effects of Social Connection and Community* (Washington, DC: U.S. Department of Health and Human Services, 2023), https://www.hhs.gov/sites/default/files/surgeon-general-social-connection-advisory.pdf.

PART VIII Living Long, Living Well

1. R.M. Ravindran and V.R. Kutty, 'Burden of Falls among Elderly Persons in India: A Systematic Review and Meta-Analysis', *The National Medical Journal of India* 34, no. 5 (2021): 295–299, https://doi.org/10.25259/NMJI_110_20.
2. 'Falls', World Health Organization, 26 April 2021, https://www.who.int/news-room/fact-sheets/detail/falls/.
3. V. Rajalakshmi, K. Philip et al., 'Prevalence and Risk Factors for Falls in Community-Dwelling Older Population in Kerala: A Cross-Sectional Study', *Heliyon* 9, no. 8 (2023), https://doi.org/10.1016/j.heliyon.2023.e18737.
4. E. Volpi, R. Nazemi, and S. Fujita, 'Muscle Tissue Changes with Aging', *Current Opinion in Clinical Nutrition & Metabolic Care* 13, no. 4 (2010): 405–410.
5. A.J. Cruz-Jentoft, G. Bahat, J. Bauer et al., 'Sarcopenia: Revised European Consensus on Definition and Diagnosis', *Age and Ageing* 48, no. 1 (2019): 16–31.
6. T.E. Howe et al., 'Exercise for Preventing and Treating Osteoporosis in Postmenopausal Women', *Cochrane Database of Systematic Reviews* 7 (2011).
7. K.D. Tipton and S.M. Phillips, 'Dietary Protein for Muscle Hypertrophy', *Nestlé Nutrition Institute Workshop Series* 76 (2013): 73–84.
8. Y. Stern et al., 'Whitepaper: Defining and Investigating Cognitive Reserve, Brain Reserve, and Brain Maintenance', *The Lancet Neurology* 19, no. 1 (2020): 70–78. https://doi.org/10.1016/S1474-4422(19)30353-8.
9. J. Verghese, R.B. Lipton, M. J. Katz et al., 'Leisure Activities and the Risk of Dementia in the Elderly', *Archives of Neurology* 60, no. 6 (2003): 2508–2516, https://doi.org/10.1001/archneur.60.6.2508.
10. N.L. Spartano et al., 'Midlife Exercise Blood Pressure, Heart Rate, and Fitness Relate to Brain Volume 2 Decades Later', *Neurology* 86, no. 14 (2016): 1313–1319.
11. S. Leonardo and F. Fregni, 'Association of Inflammation and Cognition in the Elderly: A Systematic Review and Meta-analysis', *Frontiers in Aging Neuroscience* 15 (2023): 1069439. https://doi.org/10.3389/fnagi.2023.1069439.

About the Author

Dr Nandita Iyer is a medical doctor and wellness educator with additional certifications in nutrition and mental health. She offers personalised coaching, helping individuals navigate their health journey with science-backed, practical guidance. The author of four books on healthy eating, food, and lifestyle, she has also been writing a fortnightly column for *Mint Lounge* for the past eight years. Her blog, Saffron Trail, launched in 2006, laid the foundation for her influential work in nutrition and wellness.

A lifelong learner, she is dedicated to demystifying food, health, and wellness, making evidence-based practices accessible and easy to follow. Alongside her work, she has spent over a decade training in Hindustani classical vocal music, embodying her belief in pursuing art as a path to a fulfilling life.

Originally from Mumbai, where she lived for over three decades, Nandita now calls Bengaluru home. Her holistic and science-based approach to well-being continues to inspire and empower individuals to lead healthier, more balanced lives.

You can follow her on X and on Instagram @saffrontrail.